SOCIAL POLICY, PUBLIC POLICY

Professor Meredith Edwards has spent her career as a lecturer, researcher and policy analyst. Before becoming Deputy Vice-Chancellor of the University of Canberra in 1997, she worked in several departments of the Commonwealth Public Service, including Social Security, Education and Employment, and Community Services and Health. The last four years of her public service career were spent as Deputy Secretary, Department of Prime Minister and Cabinet. **Cosmo Howard** has recently completed a study of the processes surrounding the 1994 *Working Nation* White Paper on Employment and Growth; he is currently researching the implementation of the coalition government's *Mutual Obligation Initiative* for the unemployed and undertaking a PhD in the Graduate Program in Public Policy at the Australian National University, Canberra. **Robin Miller** is a member of the Centre for Research in Public Sector Management at the University of Canberra. He was previously in the Senior Executive Service of the Australian Public Service, serving with the Department of Defence and former Industries Assistance Commission.

SOCIAL POLICY, PUBLIC POLICY

From problem to practice

Meredith Edwards
with
Cosmo Howard and Robin Miller

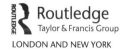

Routledge
Taylor & Francis Group

LONDON AND NEW YORK

First published 2001 by Allen & Unwin

Published 2020 by Routledge
2 Park Square, Milton Park, Abingdon, Oxon OX14 4RN
605 Third Avenue, New York, NY 10017

Routledge is an imprint of the Taylor & Francis Group, an informa business

National Library of Australia
Catloguing-in-Publication entry:

Edwards, Meredith.
    Social policy, public policy: from problems to practice.

    Bibliography.
    Includes index.
    ISBN 1 86448 948 0.

    1. Australia—Social policy. 2. Australia—Politics and government. I. Howard, Cosmo. II. Miller, Robin, 1933– .
    III. Title.

352.340994

Set in 9.5/12 pt Arrus by DOCUPRO, Canberra

ISBN-13: 9781864489484 (pbk)

Contents

Preface

The origins of this book date back more than ten years when, as a senior policy adviser, I was involved in a complex but comprehensive policy development process that led to a radical policy reform: Australia's Child Support Scheme.

Through that experience I saw the value of a systematic approach to policy development in helping to achieve desired social policy reform. It was then that I realised the value of a book of this kind to assist up-and-coming policy advisers to increase their potential for contributing to good policy processes.

The book aims to attract another group of readers: students of social and public policy. Over the past ten or so years, I have often been called on to share my policy experiences with students of public administration and public policy. This has led to lively sessions comparing what the textbooks say happens, with what my experiences suggest can actually happen. So this book is also written as a text for students, aiming to bridge theory and practice by providing both illustrative descriptive material and useful and general prescriptions through case studies.

There is little literature on how to evaluate what policy advisers do, let alone how to evaluate the processes that lead to that advice. I hope the material in this book will, therefore, assist in improving the skills of people who may wish to assess the performance of policy advisers and social policy development processes more generally.

This book has been written from the perspective of a policy adviser. Policy advisers cannot help but be affected by their own value framework, despite a reluctance to acknowledge that point. I had this to say back in 1992:

> Good policy advisers are (often) painted as people who are appropriately qualified and highly motivated, who rationally and objectively assess options as part of the policy development and advisory role. We all know that this is not true or at least that it is simplistic . . . Questions arise here about the extent to which the policy adviser can also be an advocate, at least once the Minister is of the same view. Questions also arise about whether or not value positions should be made explicit to superiors and the Minister in any assessment of the policy advice provided. (Edwards 1992:447)

Between 1983 and 1997 I was a policy adviser with a real commitment to making a difference in areas of social policy. Most of that time I was a senior public servant and worked in a central agency (Prime Minister and Cabinet) and line departments (e.g. DSS and DEET). I was a ministerial consultant for just over a year when assisting with the development of the Child Support Scheme, but (unusually for the time) worked out of DSS and for most purposes acted as a public servant.

My values were known to the people who worked with me. Those values related to wanting to address the inequities I perceived in the ways in which government policies affected certain groups of people, such as families, unemployed people, people with disabilities and, more generally, lower-income people (including children). I wanted to improve the quality of life for these people in our society. Soon after joining the bureaucracy from academia, I became aware that more equity could not easily (if at all) be achieved unless the social policy agenda was fitted into the broader and more prominent economic agenda of the time.

In each policy exercise with which I was involved, I set about providing policy advice that drew out the efficiency as well as equity implications of reform. On reflection I was probably what Yeatman (1998) calls a 'policy activist': a policy adviser strongly committed to promoting an agenda. I was fortunate to work for ministers who, in the main, were not only determined to get results but who had value systems consistent with my own. This, in my view, does not detract from providing good policy advice outside the political context:

> When a politician becomes a Minister with a particular portfolio, and discusses policy direction with the senior public officials managing

> this portfolio, Party political concerns present a series of constraints on such exchange but they do not direct its substance . . . As long as those political constraints can be worked within, the political process is subordinated to the policy process. (Yeatman 1998: 22)

There are obvious advantages in having a major 'player' tell it as it was from the 'inside'. But there is also a real limitation in that no one individual can see the whole process. Although I was a public servant and, for a short time, a ministerial consultant, I was never a politician or lobbyist. The book shows my perspective. There is always the bias that a player can bring in telling her side of the story.

Another bias is that I was more involved in the development of policy than in its implementation and so can tell fewer inside tales of the latter. Partly to counter this, I held discussions in 1998–99 with some key players in each case, and organised retrospective workshops where many of the players came together and reminisced; some quotations from these various discussions are given in boxes. The enlisting of co-authors to research and draft and comment on chapters—people who were not players in the cases chosen—also helped to counter potential bias.

It should be emphasised that there are many public servants who have considerably more experience than I have who could have written (and may still write) a book of this kind. I happened to be one who has left the public service and had an interest in telling the story from my perspective. I hope others with more to offer than I will, in the future, share their experiences.

Case studies form the centrepiece of this book. They are based on public documents for the period 1983 to 1996, but go beyond those documents and rely on the experiences of the author, assisted by journal entries made during those years (usually entered at weekends). They include a list of players mentioned in the text as well as a chronology to assist navigation through each chapter.

The particular cases in this book have been chosen because, working from within the bureaucracy, I was involved in the policy development process in each case. The value of the 'practitioner' telling it as she saw it, is to provide some insights across stages in the policy framework, insights into what is often otherwise seen as a 'black box' (Waller 1992: 443). Personal experience provides a glimpse of what policy participants actually do, and is something on which little has yet been written (see Colebatch 1998: 100). It is for this reason, rather than as mere indulgence, that I have inserted boxed entries from my journal, presented with minimal editing, when these seem to illustrate my point.

Acknowledgements

Many people were most generous with their time, and so helped make this book possible. I am grateful to all of them.

First and most importantly, I am grateful for the continued support of my co-authors, Cosmo Howard and Robin Miller. Cosmo was responsible for the first draft of Chapter 5; he also challenged my conceptual thinking, especially for Chapter 1. Robin was responsible for the first draft of Chapter 2 and, with an initial start from Chloe Flutter with interviews and drafting, for the completion of the first draft of Chapter 4. My thanks go to the senior public servants and others who were players in the development of policies which the case studies describe and who helped me in my task; also to those who pooled their memories with mine in discussions. The (then) DSS helped fund the first workshop at which the book's outline was discussed and the Child Support Agency provided assistance with the workshop of child support players.

The University of Canberra, through its Vice-Chancellor, Don Aitkin, was generous in its financial support for my research, permitting me to provide payment to a range of people to save my time. Apart from the co-authors, I was able to gain the excellent editing services of Venetia Somerset, who also helped me with a first draft of Chapter 3. Typing and administrative support was ably provided by both Ros Tassaker and Gayna Green. Amanda Lumsden, Dr Kate Burton and Betty Nathan gave some last-minute and much-needed assistance.

My good friend Doug Cocks gave many valuable comments on all chapters of the book. Bruce Chapman, a major player in two of the cases, also gave most useful comments and support, as did Alan Abrahart, Michael Keating, Allen Mawer and Chris Robinson. I wish to give heartfelt thanks to John Iremonger of Allen & Unwin, who never failed to encourage me. My family and friends deserve special thanks for their tolerance; through the process of producing this book, alongside other demands, I learnt how high can be the 'opportunity cost' of not spending time with those I cherish.

Meredith Edwards
Canberra, August 2000

Glossary

AUSTUDY	An educational allowance for secondary and tertiary students aged 16 and over, providing means-tested income support for students engaged in approved full-time secondary and tertiary studies. (CEO 1993: 212)
Batch processing	Processing forms in lots rather than singly, e.g. tax forms.
Beveridge curve	The relationship between the level of unemployment and unfilled job vacancies: as unemployment rises the competition for vacancies coming on to the market increases and the number of unfilled vacancies falls. (CEO 1993: 212)
Budget deficit	Situation in which government expenditure exceeds revenue.
Cabinet	A group of senior ministers, responsible for a government's major policy decisions. (Bridgman and Davis 2000: 169)
Cabinet memorandum	A document for Cabinet prepared by officials (usually an IDC) for discussion and decision.
Cabinet submission	A document for Cabinet prepared by a Minister or Ministers for discussion and decision.
Case management	Mechanism to provide individualised assistance to unemployed or other category of

	person requiring assistance; often involves services from several government programs.
Caucus	All members of parliamentary Labor Party who meet to discuss tactics or set policies.
Central agency	A department or office within a department responsible for policy, economic or personnel coordination across government. Central policy agencies are usually those supporting the head of government, the Treasurer or the Minister for Finance. (Bridgman and Davis 2000: 170)
Child maintenance payments	Amount paid by non-custodial parent to custodial parent for support of child(ren); determined by a court.
Child support	Administratively-based system of child maintenance payments.
Commonwealth Ombudsman	Organisation assessing complaints from the public against decisions and actions of government, the bureaucracy and some private contractors providing public services.
Competitive neutrality	Ensuring that neither private operators nor public agencies are advantaged when competing for the right to provide public services.
Consultation	A structured process to seek, and respond to, views about a policy issue from relevant interest groups or individuals, or the community generally. (Bridgman and Davis 2000: 170)
Contracting out	Provision of goods or services, that usually were previously provided internally, by one organisation to another, under a contract and on a commercial basis.
Dole bludgers	Term implying disapproval of recipients of unemployment benefit.
Efficiency	Extent to which inputs are minimised for given level of outputs.
Electoral cycle	Time between elections which can affect government decision-making.
Equity	Equal treatment of people in similar circumstances (horizontal) or differential treatment of people in different circumstances (vertical), as in income taxation systems which normally tax people on higher incomes proportionately more than people on lower incomes.

Evaluation	A process for examining the worth of a program, by measuring outputs and outcomes, and comparing these with targets. (Bridgman and Davis 2000: 171)
Ex-nuptial children	Children born out of marriage.
Expenditure Review Committee	Key Cabinet Committee responsible for consideration of budget savings and expenditure measures, across all government agencies.
External environment	Broader context within which policy decisions need to be made.
Fiscal	Pertaining to public revenue, especially taxation.
GDP	Gross domestic product; a measure of a country's total net output.
Green paper	Government discussion paper usually with issues, options and sometimes proposals as a basis for public consultation, typically developed before a white paper.
Gridlock	Situation where decision-making cannot be progressed due to conflicting interests.
Higher education sector	Education provided by the university sector.
Honest broker	Person recognised as being able to give disinterested help in resolving conflicts of interest.
Hypothecating revenue	Earmarking government revenue for a particular purpose.
Implementation	The process of converting a policy decision into action. (Bridgman and Davis 2000: 172)
Income-contingent loans scheme	Scheme in which loan repayments are dependent upon the income level of the recipient.
Income support policies	Policies affecting the distribution of resources to individuals or families usually designed to assist certain groups achieve particular minimum income levels.
Income test	The way in which income support payments are assessed when the recipient receives private income, for example from part-time work. (CEO 1993: 214)
Institutional memory	Knowledge of organisational procedures and histories retained through time.
Interdepartmental committee (IDC)	Forum in which representatives of several government agencies meet to formulate policy advice or agree on program implementation.

Job compact	A mutual obligation agreement between the government and long-term unemployed people on job-seeking and gaining a job.
Jobs Education and Training (JET)	A program for sole-parent pensioners administered jointly by (then) DSS, DEET and the Department of Health, Housing, Local Government and Community Services which took into account employment, childcare and other needs of the parent.
Jobs levy	An income tax surcharge to finance costs of employment programs for long-term unemployed people.
Jobs Skills	A work experience and training program with fully subsidised placements in the local government and community sectors. (CEO 1993: 215)
Job Start	A wage subsidy scheme whereby employers receive(d) subsidised payments as an incentive for employing disadvantaged job seekers. (CEO 1993: 215)
Labour market program	Government-funded assistance for the unemployed including training wage subsidies for employers and job assistance. (CEO 1993)
Legislation	Law made by parliament or by another person or body under a delegation by parliament. (Bridgman and Davis 2000: 173)
Line department	A government department responsible for delivery of specific public services to the community.
Lobbyists	People seeking to influence government decisions.
Longitudinal study	Data or research project tracking changes over time.
Long-term unemployment	Unemployed continuously for more than a year. (CEO 1993: 216)
Managerialist approach in public administration	Adopting management practices commonly found in the private sector, into the public sector, e.g. strategic management, results focus, devolution of decision making, commercialisation of certain activities, etc.
New Start	An active framework for assistance to unemployed people combining income support, activity-based systematic client contact and

labour market program assistance. (CEO 1993)

Non-custodial parent
The parent who does not have the day-to-day care of his/her child(ren).

Organisation for Economic Cooperation and Development (OECD)
An organisation of industrialised countries which seeks to promote coordination of economic and social policies between its members.

Outcomes
The impact of a policy decision or program by which program effectiveness can be judged.

Outputs
The product or services produced by a person or program.

Parliamentary Joint Select Committee
Committee of both houses of Parliament addressing a specific as distinct from an ongoing issue.

Pay as you Earn (PAYE)
Taxation system in which tax payments are deducted from wages or salaries at source.

Perverse incentives
Incentives that have opposite effects from those intended.

Policy analysis
Analysis of a policy problem, designed to state the nature of the problem and lead to options for addressing the issue; or analysis of government's action, designed to discern the underlying policy choices of that government. (Bridgman and Davis 2000: 174)

Policy entrepreneurship
Active promotion of a policy idea by a public servant.

Political opportunism
Taking advantage of an unexpected situation to achieve a political goal.

Portfolio
A department or group of agencies for which a Minister is responsible.

Positive spillover effects
Beneficial side effects.

Post-hoc rationalisation
Justifying a decision already taken.

Purchaser–provider arrangement
Organisational arrangement which separates the purchaser of goods or services from the provider of those goods or services. Separation may occur within a single agency or between agencies.

Reciprocal obligation
A situation where parties are seen to have obligations to each other.

Regressivity	Having a disproportionate impact on lower income groups.
Retention rates	Proportion of students completing a nominated year of school.
Revenue clawback	Monies collected to wholly or partially repay government payments to individuals, e.g. the Higher Education Contributions Scheme.
Single youth allowance	A uniform level of payment to all young people irrespective of whether they are students, disabled or unemployed.
Social policy	Policies designed to redress inequities and encourage active participation in the labour market.
Stakeholders	People or groups with an interest in the outcomes of decisions or programs.
Strategic planning	A process of deciding how an organisation's major goals are to be implemented.
Summit	Meeting of stakeholder groups to make collective recommendations to government about key national issues, e.g. the Tax Summit.
Tertiary sector	Education and training provided by both the university and vocational education sectors.
Think-tank	Group of people charged with developing policy ideas and options around particular issues.
Training wage	Payment below market rates for individuals who are being trained in the workplace.
Unemployment	As defined by the ABS, a person is unemployed when he or she is aged 15 and over, is without work but is available for work in the reference week; and has actively looked for full- or part-time work in the last four weeks.
Voucher system	System which pays students a sum of money to be used at the educational institution of their choice. This method determines the funding to be allocated to each institution.
Westminster model	System of government in which it is presumed that there is separation of power between the executive, the legislature and judicial arms of government.
White Paper	Statement of a government's policy intention in a particular area, traditionally printed on white bond paper. (Bridgman and Davis 2000: 174)

Abbreviations

ABS	Australian Bureau of Statistics
ABSEC	Aboriginal Secondary Assistance Scheme
ABSTUDY	Aboriginal Study Assistance Scheme
ACCESS	Australian Contribution to the Cost of Education for Students Scheme
ACOSS	Australian Council of Social Services
ACTU	Australian Council of Trade Unions
AFR	*Australian Financial Review*
AG	Attorney-General
AGs	Attorney-General's Department
AIC	Assistance for Isolated Children
AIFS	Australian Institute of Family Studies
ALP	Australian Labor Party
AMEP-LA	Adult Migrant Education Program—Living Allowance
ANAO	Australian National Audit Office
ANOP	Australian National Opinion Polls
ANU	Australian National University
ARC	Australian Research Council
ATO	Australian Taxation Office
AVCC	Australian Vice-Chancellors' Committee
CEO	Committee on Employment Opportunities
CES	Commonwealth Employment Service
CSA	Child Support Agency
CSCG	Child Support Consultative Group
CSEAG	Child Support Evaluation Advisory Group

CTEC	Commonwealth Tertiary Education Commission
DEET	Department of Employment, Education and Training (July 1987–March 1996)
DEETYA	Department of Employment, Education, Training and Youth Affairs (from March 1996; now DETYA)
DEYA	Department of Education and Youth Affairs (March 1983–December 1984; then became Department of Education alongside Department of Employment and Industrial Relations until July 1987)
DSS	Department of Social Security
EPAD	Economic and Policy Analysis Division
ERC	Expenditure Review Committee
FLC	Family Law Council
GDP	Gross Domestic Product
HEAC	Higher Education Administration Charge
HEC	Higher Education Council
HECS	Higher Education Contribution Scheme
HR	House of Representatives
HRSC	House of Representatives Standing Committee
IDC	interdepartmental committee
IT	information technology
IYY	International Youth Year
JET	Jobs, Education and Training
LTU	long-term unemployed/unemployment
MA	Maintenance Allowance
NBEET	National Board of Employment, Education and Training
NCP	non-custodial parent
NZ LPCS	New Zealand Liable Parent Contribution Scheme
OECD	Organization of Economic Cooperation and Development
ORR	Office of Regulation Review
OYA	Office of Youth Affairs
PM&C	(Department of) Prime Minister and Cabinet
PMO	Prime Minister's Office
SAS	Secondary Allowances Scheme
SJP	Social Justice Project
SMH	*Sydney Morning Herald*
SPRC	Social Policy Research Centre
SWPS	Social Welfare Policy Secretariat
TEAS	Tertiary Education Assistance Scheme
TFYAA	Task Force on Youth Allowance Administration
UB	Unemployment Benefit
VCES	Veterans' Children Education Scheme
YACA	Youth Affairs Council of Australia

Chapter One

Introducing policy processes

This is a book about government policy processes: it examines the way government ministers and public servants, as well as experts such as academics and others in the community, work together to develop policy from its conception through to its practice.

Ministers are the ultimate policy-makers but government officials can help them immeasurably, not only by advising on policy but also by being aware of the capacity of the policy development process to contribute to the policy objectives of their political masters. Even in the midst of political chaos, there is a part that public servants can play by being conscious of the value of being as rigorous as possible in how they do their work, individually and with others.

Recently the Australian public sector has seen major changes, particularly increased activity in contracting the private sector to take on business previously undertaken within government agencies. Core functions of government have been under serious review. One core function remaining, however, is policy advice and development. In the environment of the 'contracting state', there are, I hope, some insights in this book not only for public servants and political advisers, but also for those in the private and community sectors who deal with government.

A recent impetus for this book was the publication, in late 1999 (a second edition appeared in 2000), of a most useful 'how-to' book by Peter Bridgman and Glyn Davis, *Australian Policy Handbook*. It offers a possible path through the complexities of decision-making and a practical guide to stages in the policy process. The purpose of this book is to provide some concrete examples, through case studies, to accompany Bridgman and Davis's generalisations, and in this way to be a complementary textbook. It is not the purpose of this book to develop a new theoretical structure on how policy is or should be developed, although it is hoped that the case studies provided may assist scholars in further refining their models of the policy process. Bailey's observation about the interaction of scholars' works and practitioners' experience is relevant here:

> The information that practitioners own is needed by scholars to develop and test theories, which can then be applied by practitioners to improve the practice of public administration and by scholars both in further theory development and for the teaching of public managers. (1994: 190)

While the four cases presented in Chapters 2–5 arise out of Australian Commonwealth experience, and under a Labor government, their lessons, on reflection, are just as relevant for other levels of government as well as for governments of various persuasions, both here and overseas.

GOOD POLICY PROCESSES: A POLICY DEVELOPMENT FRAMEWORK

The purpose of putting effort into good policy development processes is to ensure that as far as possible, good outcomes emerge. Michael Keating has argued that 'a good policy process is a vital underpinning of good policy development. Of course, good process does not necessarily guarantee a good policy outcome, but the risks of bad process leading to a bad outcome are very much higher' (1996: 63).

There is no universal answer to the much-debated question of what is good policy or a good policy outcome—what is meant by 'good' is inherently subjective. But one expected response is that good policy is policy that achieves its objectives as set by the decision-makers. This could be a single minister or a group of ministers, such as Cabinet. If the objectives are not clear, obviously it is hard to judge the achievements of a policy process. It could also be argued that good policy can be expected to be durable and sustainable—so long, of course, as external circumstances do not overtake the original objectives of the policy, which does happen. Support from a wide range of players for the values and objectives that lie behind a policy would be expected. Without that support, policy can be undermined in its implementation or in other ways by lobbyists and others, and hence have little chance of being sustainable.

It is a key premise of this book, therefore, that good policy processes are necessary in most instances to ensure good outcomes in terms of achieving objectives, although they may not be sufficient on their own.

At a more basic level, a good policy development process will be rigorous and will broadly follow an organising framework (such as the rigour found in processes followed by the Commonwealth Government around regulation development [ORR 1998] and also by the Ralph Review [1998]). Several broad policy frameworks have appeared in public administration literature over the last 50 years, with refinements along the way (e.g. May and Wildavsky 1978; Hogwood and Gunn 1984; Davis et al. 1993; Edwards 1993; Hawke 1993; Howlett and Ramesh 1995; Colebatch 1998). Much of that literature debates the relevance of what has become known as the 'rational model'—a scientific approach to finding a solution to a problem (but see the well-known essay by Lindblom [1959]). In the literature the alternative to 'rational' is not 'irrational' but 'incremental', a process by which decisions are made by building on current policies 'step-by-step and by small degrees' (Lindblom 1959: 81). (For further discussion, see Bridgman and Davis 2000: 64).

Policy environments are full of complexities, usually involving a diverse range of players coming from different perspectives and spawning a host of unexpected events. It is therefore very unlikely that circumstances would permit anything approaching classical rationality in the decision-making process. It is not proposed to enter the somewhat sterile debate about whether or not the policy processes described in this book were 'rational' or not. Rather, the starting point for this book is that despite the complexities of the real world, a systematic approach to policy development can deliver significant benefits of order and process in addressing policy problems (see also Bridgman and Davis 2000: 48). An analogy here is the reliance of an organisation on strategic planning processes to improve performance, despite the lack of control of the organisation over the external environment.

THE POLICY FRAMEWORK

In the context of policy development, a rigorous approach is commonly referred to as the 'policy cycle' model (Bridgman and Davis 2000), or as I prefer to call it, a 'policy development framework'.

The framework I have found most useful in practice, especially when chairing government interdepartmental committees (IDCs), and which I have used with students of public policy in an attempt to encourage good practice, contains stages similar to those in Bridgman and Davis (Edwards 1993). What follows is that framework with slight modification to fit in with the wording used by Bridgman and Davis.

A modified Bridgman and Davis framework for policy development

- Identify issues
  - problem defined
  - problem articulated
- Policy analysis
  - collect relevant data and information
  - clarify objectives and resolve key questions
  - develop options and proposals
- Undertake consultation
- Move towards decisions
- Implement
- Evaluate

Each case study is organised around the above approach. Regardless of the names given to the various stages in the cycle or framework, *the purpose is to gain the benefit of breaking up the policy process into clear steps in order to manage the complexities of developing policy in a systematic and rigorous manner.* As Howlett and Ramesh put it:

> The advantage of employing the cycle model is that it facilitates the understanding of the public policy process by breaking it into sub-processes, each of which can be investigated alone or in terms of its relationship to the other stages of the cycle. This allows study of individual cases, a comparative study of a series of cases, or study of one or many stages of one or several cases. The model's greatest virtue, however, is its empirical orientation which enables analysis of a wide range of different factors at work at the various stages. (1995: 198)

THE POLICY STAGES EXPLAINED

Identifying the issues is the initial stage when an issue demands government attention and where the nature of the problem is clarified and articulated. The empirical evidence is that commonly the policy process is initiated from within government (Howlett and Ramesh 1995: 105; Hall et al. 1986). A key question to address early on, therefore, in the context of the case studies to follow, is how the problem got on the agenda and how it was articulated. Until there is broad acceptance of the nature of the policy problem, it is difficult to move on. This point is put well by Parsons:

> We may all agree what an issue is but disagree as to what exactly the problem is, and therefore what policy should be pursued. If we see people sleeping on the streets as a problem of vagrancy, then the policy response may be framed in terms of law enforcement and policing. (Hill 1997: 115, quoting Parsons 1995: 87)

Senior ministers can be heavily involved in articulating the problem and ensuring that there is broad enough acceptance of the issue to move towards its resolution. Here lobby groups and the media can play a significant part in putting the problem on the agenda and informing the public about it. And senior bureaucrats will try to influence the policy agendas of their ministers according to their own priorities. If they are politically astute, they will take into account how crowded and competing those agendas are.

The *policy analysis* stage follows. Policy analysis can be quite complex. It is useful in my experience to divide the analysis into the three elements identified above:

- collecting relevant data and undertaking relevant research
- clarifying objectives if needed, and identifying areas of disagreement as key questions requiring guidance from policy-makers on direction before moving on to
- developing options and proposals for reform.

Some questions addressed in discussing this stage of the policy framework include: Where did the data and research come from and what was its significance in affecting the identification of the problem, the issues and the options? How did key players interact and how were areas of disagreement identified? When and how were they resolved? At what stage were options developed and by whom and in what forums? Were criteria used to assess the options, and if so, what were they? What can be understood about bureaucratic politics from these events?

The next identified stage in policy analysis is *consultation*. Consultation can be formal or informal, and continuous or episodic. It can therefore occur at any, perhaps all stages in developing policy. What happened in each case? When did formal consultation occur in the cycle and why? How was it undertaken and how was that decision made? To what extent did consultation lead to policy refinement and affect policy decisions? In other words, policy debates that take place outside government often lead to political sensitivity on certain proposals and hence action (Dalton et al. 1996). While consultation should and usually does take place throughout the policy development process, and good judgment is required on what type of consultation is needed, formal consultation seems most appropriate when some key issues and/or options are on the table and before final decisions are made.

This book illustrates what Bridgman and Davis call the 'consult-ation diamond': earlier and later stages in policy development tend to be kept within the public sector; it is in the middle stage that there is greater public participation 'as assumptions are tested . . . [and t]he foundations are laid for community acceptance of the ultimate policy, and additional data gathered' (2000: 78).

Ultimately, following refinement of original proposals, *policy decisions* emerge.

Major decisions emerged as a result of Cabinet deliberations in the cases covered in the following chapters. This part of each chapter tells the story around the making of policy decisions, the extent to which there was difficulty reaching a decision, the role of key players, and the unexpected political and other hurdles.

The most undervalued part of the policy process is what happens after Cabinet decisions have been made, that is, the *implementation* of policy (see Gunn 1978; Colebatch and Ryan 1995; Colebatch 1998). Colebatch identifies some of the reasons implementation falters:

> Other studies of implementation . . . found a number of . . . causes for policies not being implemented: the original decision was ambigu-ous; the policy direction conflicted with other policies; it was not seen as a high priority; there were insufficient resources to carry it out; it provoked conflict with other significant players; the target group proved hard to reach; the things that were done did not have the expected impact; attention shifted to other problems etc.
> (Colebatch 1998: 56)

There is certainly evidence of this in the following chapters. The cases attempt to ask questions such as: What were the issues that arose in implementation and how were they resolved? How impor-tant were time and resource constraints? To what extent were they anticipated in the policy development process? In what ways did implementation processes, including the development of legislation, lead to a movement away from original policy intentions?

Finally, *evaluation* of the policy occurs, which can lead back to policy revisions. In the four cases studied, the evaluation objective was to assess the extent to which the policy objectives originally set were actually met and met efficiently. Questions asked here include: How successful was the policy and how was it judged? What reviews were undertaken and were they external or internal to the department or government? Why? How important was politics in the process?

The evaluation stage, as a few of the following cases show, is not necessarily a neutral, technical exercise but can be as politically charged as any of the other policy development phases. To understand the evaluation stage, it is therefore important to consider also who initiates the evaluation, why, and how it is organised—specifically, who undertakes it and with what terms of reference.

There are limitations in relying on the policy cycle/framework construct (see Bridgman and Davis 2000: 26). Most important in the context of this book, while this type of framework may be appropriate for fundamental policy changes (see Dror 1964; Edwards 1996), it may not be appropriate for other policy changes, for example incremental changes to policy in a budget context. In addition, there can be traps in assuming that there is a common set of values, or objectives, among key players or decision-makers. Discussed in this section are the qualifications that need to be made to any assumption of a linear progression from identification of the problem, or issue identification stage, through to obtaining an outcome.

Nevertheless, seen for what it is, a simplifying analytical construct, the policy framework can serve as a bridge between some ideal of process and the practice. It can be a most useful tool in pursuing success for a policy position.

THE 'POLICY DANCE'

> A policy cycle cannot capture the full ebb and flow of a sophisticated policy debate, nor does it accommodate fully the value-laden world of politics. Experience shows that the normative sequence is easily disrupted. The policy dance is sometimes seemingly random movements rather than choreographed order. (Bridgman and Davis 2000: 31)

Each policy reform analysed in this book went through each stage in the policy development framework. Unless key stages in the policy process are reached, it is difficult to move on towards solutions. It appears, for instance, that it is necessary to identify the problem and articulate it clearly to the point where it has broad recognition among the stakeholders that count, before it is possible to move towards a policy solution.

On the other hand, a noticeable feature in the cases that follow was that stages were sometimes revisited; in other words there was some backwards as well as forwards movement across stages. In this sense the process could be said to be iterative. In some cases it could be said to be inefficient (if not irrational) to backtrack; in other cases backtracking appeared to be the only way through to a solution, as when, for political reasons, following lobby group and media attention, the Child Support Scheme was phased in and implemented in two stages.

In addition, although time was spent on each stage in the policy development framework, the stages sometimes overlapped: for example, overlap between policy analysis and consultation, which can be useful in obtaining consensus on options. An interesting observation from the cases is the relationship between problems and solutions, which is also a conclusion noted in a book on British social policy case studies:

> There is a complicated relationship between problems and solutions which is itself one of the important explanations of why certain policies emerge. Logically, the identification and analysis of a problem precedes proposals for a remedy, but in reality the sequence is less tidy . . . The very fact that remedies are attractive and available may advance the priority of certain problems to which they can be applied. (Hall et al. 1986: 490)

The general conclusion here is that even though there can be forwards and backwards 'policy dances' and overlap of stages, unless each policy stage is addressed in policy reform, it is unlikely that any major policy proposal will have a chance of being implemented.

PROCESSES, PLAYERS AND POLITICS

> In all policy development work in which I have been involved, a major issue in providing policy advice to the Minister is to decide how to handle strategically the policy process. This includes dealing with potential opposition . . . for example, should there be an inter-departmental committee . . .? Is so, at what stage? If not, how are other relevant departmental players to be involved? Is an external review more appropriate? Outcomes can depend as much on high quality advice about the process to be followed as on particular options. (Edwards 1992: 448)

While the policy framework approach can contribute to reaching and understanding good policy outcomes, it needs to be seen as just one of several possible levels of analysis of the policy process (Howard 1998), sitting alongside other factors that also assist in explaining what happens. Colebatch usefully distinguishes between the vertical dimension to policy development (the policy framework as described here) and other factors, which he describes as horizontal:

> The horizontal dimension is concerned with relationships among policy participants in different organizations—that is, outside the line of hierarchical authority. It recognizes that policy work takes place across organizational boundaries as well as within them, and consists in the structure of understandings and commitments among participants in different organizations as well as the hierarchical transmission of authorized decisions within any one organization. (Colebatch 1998: 39)

This book takes a somewhat broader interpretation of 'horizontal' factors. The cases in the following chapters illustrate some important factors that affect successful outcomes at some, if not every, stage of the policy framework. They demonstrate the value of the role of the broader economic, social and political context and how the problem is placed within that (such as the size of the budget deficit or the stage in the electoral cycle); they show the value of carefully choosing organisational processes and structures, as well as key players, and the value of their networks; and they show the scope for 'political opportunism' and policy entrepreneurship. The role of politics is, of course, forever present and, as can be expected, is ultimately paramount in affecting policy outcomes (May 1991).

A common thread throughout the cases is the careful consideration given to the organisational structures within which much of the policy analysis occurred. In one theoretical view of the Westminster model, departments advise and Cabinet coordinates policy through processes such as the budget (Painter and Carey 1979). This is not necessarily a realistic description of the process for complex and interdependent cross-portfolio policy-making, which demands that the relationships between policy areas be explored and assessed before ministers take decisions.

The role of academics as players is another strong theme throughout the following chapters. Academics are players in the sense of producing relevant research to feed a policy process and also, at times, to give it direction. The cases also show the role the media can play—both positive and negative, and especially the former.

The value of informal networks of key players at each stage in the policy development process has been noted in the literature and also appears in the following cases. Dalton makes this point well:

> Because people in organizations are involved in making policy, then the full range of organizational strategies are brought to bear. In a shadow behind the formal process, there is often a series of phone

calls, lunches, breakfasts, media leaks, meetings of both a regular and irregular kind. (Dalton et al. 1996: 107)

Much that happens in developing policy is out of the control of any one player—whether public servant, academic, lobbyist, or other. The electoral cycle can play a large part in determining what items get on the agenda and when and whether they are pursued past a certain point; sensitivities in the electorate at any time, or even within a party, can stop issues emerging or stall their development. Even ministers can find their policy agendas thwarted if, for example, other ministerial colleagues, especially the Prime Minister, are not on side. Certain items at times claim dominance in the political agenda; this can thwart attempts at promoting other competing items unless they tie in with that dominant concern, for example fiscal responsibility. But wherever a player sits in the policy process, inside or outside government, opportunities for advancing policy reforms do arise. When opportunity does arise, it is useful to understand the broader framework of policy development and at what stage or stages a player can take an effective part.

THE CASE STUDIES

Case studies have not been used extensively in Australian texts on public or social policy (but see Dalton et al. 1996). The reason for their use is to observe and assess the public policy 'laboratory'. This can be of benefit to practitioners, especially when the cases are based on the experience of their colleagues (Bailey in White and Adams 1994: 189). And cases placed in the context of a policy framework can add detail to more abstract policy texts or policy manuals.

The four cases selected for this book span the period 1983–96. They have much in common: they all centre on policy initiatives that led on to the achievement of radical policy reforms; all show a concerted effort to obtain a 'policy breakthrough' in attempting long-term structural reform. They all started with a fairly simple idea: a single youth allowance, a child support levy, a graduate tax and a job compact. They all relate to social policy reform where both efficiency and equity objectives needed to be met; and as will be demonstrated in each case, there was extensive use of research materials, often especially commissioned and in each case involving academic researchers.

All of the selected cases involve complexity in policy processes and show what was achievable with a sometimes exceptionally comprehensive use of processes, despite the odds. But each case is distinct in what it teaches about policy processes and why each radical policy succeeded. A by-product is that the cases, taken together, provide a useful history of major social policy reforms from the mid-1980s to the mid-1990s.

Finally, this is a book that was written to illustrate characteristics of good policy development. It is not a purpose of this book to provide case studies of how policy development went wrong and why, although some obvious deficiencies in policy process are covered. There is certainly a need for a separate book on 'bad' policy processes and what can be learned from them (Dunleavy 1995). Perhaps someone will be inspired to follow this book with something of that kind.

OUTLINE OF THE BOOK

The following chapters use the modified Bridgman and Davis framework to analyse four major social policy studies.

Chapter 2 deals with policy developed between 1983 and 1987 to simplify the existing youth allowance structure. It culminated in a new set of arrangements for students and young unemployed, with what was named AUSTUDY replacing several existing educational allowances.

Chapter 3 deals with the Child Support Scheme developed between 1985 and 1989, concentrating on the policy development and implementation of the first of the two stages of that scheme.

Chapter 4 presents the policy development process from the end of 1987 to early in 1989 concerning the introduction of the Higher Education Contribution Scheme (HECS).

Chapter 5 presents policy processes between 1993 and 1995 which culminated in the budget paper *Working Nation* (P. Keating 1994).

The structure of each of the case chapters is similar. Each starts by setting the historical and 'bigger picture' context in which the particular policy issue under scrutiny was raised. Before presenting a stage-by-stage treatment of policy development, there is a discussion of the main players, their networks and the relevant organisational structures.

The final chapter draws out some generalisations from the cases and suggests some future directions which I hope will lead to better policy processes practised by governments in years ahead.

INCOME SUPPORT FOR YOUNG PEOPLE
CHRONOLOGY OF EVENTS MARCH 1983 TO JANUARY 1987

1983

March Hawke Government elected. Ryan appointed Minister for Education and Youth Affairs. Wilenski appointed by Ryan as Secretary of her department (DEYA). OYA transferred to it.

May IDC established to develop comprehensive approach to youth policy, including youth allowances.

June OECD invited to report on Australia's youth policies. DEYA published background paper. Wilenski paper on youth income support.

October OECD team visited Australia and conducted interviews.

1984

February OYA/SWPS published paper, *Income Support for Young People*.

March Special meeting of Youth Ministers' Council to consider youth income support, OECD report and Commonwealth–State cooperation in youth affairs.

April IDC on Youth Policies started meetings on income support.

August Treasurer announced a review of youth income support arrangements.

1985

January IDC memorandum to Cabinet on youth income support issues and options.

February–April Dawkins presented a series of submissions to Cabinet on youth income options.

March Dawkins established TFYAA to simplify delivery of services.

April Youth Policy Taskforce established in OYA to draft government statement on youth policy for 1985/86 Budget.

August Government announced a new youth allowance structure in a White Paper, *The Commonwealth Government's Strategy for Young People*.

1986

March TFYAA submitted reported to ministers.

August Dawkins published paper to accompany the 1986/87 Budget.

1987

January AUSTUDY replaced TEAS and SAS.

January Assistance for Isolated Children (AIC), Adult Migrant Education Program—Living Allowance (AMEP-LA), Maintenance Allowance for refugee wards (MA) and Veterans' Children Education Scheme (VCES) incorporated into common allowances structure.

Chapter TWO

Income support for young people: The search for a single allowance

Considerable efforts have been made by Australian governments over the past fifteen to twenty years to encourage young people to better their education. One important initiative of the 1980s was the introduction of a scheme to become known as AUSTUDY—the subject of this case study. The main purpose of AUSTUDY was to provide financial assistance to young people to encourage them to complete their secondary education and gain a tertiary education. The assistance was provided through living allowances and enabled students to study full-time. Educational allowances previously paid to young people were below the Unemployment Benefit (UB) level, with the result that many chose to join the workforce or become unemployed rather than continue their education. Under AUSTUDY, living allowances were comparable to UB, thus removing the previous financial disincentive to study. Administratively, the introduction of AUSTUDY involved a major restructuring of the previous programs of income support for young people, namely UB, the Tertiary Education Assistance Scheme (TEAS) and the Secondary Allowance Scheme (SAS).

AUSTUDY began operating in January 1987 and continued until 1998, when it was largely replaced by the Youth Allowance. AUSTUDY reforms resulted in a simpler structure of allowances than had previously existed. Thus AUSTUDY replaced a complex and inconsistent structure of living allowances that had varied with the types of activity undertaken by the recipients, with a structure more related to the age of a young person.

This chapter tells the story of how AUSTUDY began, using the policy framework approach outlined in Chapter 1. It focuses on the period 1983–87, when the policies that led to AUSTUDY were initially developed and introduced through specific measures in the Labor Government's 1985/86 Budget (see Chronology). In essence there was a policy initiation phase in 1983, a research and development phase under Minister Ryan into 1984, and a more political phase under Minister Dawkins into 1985, followed by implementation in 1986 and subsequent evaluation.

One reason an examination of AUSTUDY is interesting is that the subject of income support for young people is currently topical in the new millennium. The education and training of young people is still an important public issue; and youth unemployment is still a serious problem, though not to the extent it was in the early 1980s. Some of the equity and dependency issues that figured prominently in the discussion of youth income support in the 1980s arose as the Youth Allowance was developed and put into effect in the second half of the 1990s.

AUSTUDY is also interesting as a case history because it is a good example of how professional research and analysis can be brought to bear on the making of public policy in a fairly comprehensive policy development process. Research and analysis were undertaken both inside and outside government, and much of this was published. It is an important case study for another reason also: it was an early demonstration of how a very contentious policy issue could be resolved by major structural reform. For that to occur, ministers needed to get actively involved, alongside their staff and other relevant players—something that was not common at the time.

'The youth income support exercise was a relatively early case study of a profound shift in the policy formulation process, especially the growing direct involvement of Ministers, Ministerial staff, lobbyists and academics'. (Vic Rogers, letter to author, 1999)

It might be claimed that, on the face of it, AUSTUDY was a success and for that reason alone is worthy of study. By the second half of the 1990s a much higher proportion of young people were continuing their education beyond secondary school than had been the case about a decade earlier. Since such an outcome was one of the goals of AUSTUDY, some might infer that it was a result of

AUSTUDY. But an assessment of AUSTUDY in this way would be simplistic since it is hard to disentangle which policy had what effect; governments typically address particular problems with a range of policies, and a great many factors can affect how these policies work out in practice. Issues that arise in trying to evaluate AUSTUDY are addressed later in this chapter.

HISTORY AND CONTEXT

The ideas behind most policies often have a longer history than is generally recognised. The value for a practitioner of knowing the history of a policy and its underlying ideas lies not only in the broader understanding and perspectives this brings but also in possible economies of effort when it is discovered that the wheel does not have to be reinvented.

The history of youth income support in Australia can be traced back at least to 1974, when parliament passed the Student Assistance Bill 'to produce a revolution of access to education' (Hansard, HR, 1973: 2067). The bill provided for various forms of income support such as SAS and TEAS, through which full-time students, in their last two years at school, or at universities and other tertiary institutions, were eligible for means-tested living allowances.

The Labor Opposition, intent on winning the next election, was putting youth issues firmly on the political agenda by the early 1980s. In March 1981 the shadow minister for education, John Dawkins, raised for discussion in parliament as a matter of public importance 'The failure of the Government to provide adequate support for students in secondary and tertiary education' (Hansard, HR, 1981: 420). Dawkins was Minister Assisting the Prime Minister on Youth Affairs from December 1984 to July 1987, and subsequently the Minister for Employment, Education and Training from July 1987 to December 1991, and he became a key figure in the policy processes examined in this chapter.

In his speech to parliament, Dawkins claimed that the Minister for Education was 'presiding over the deliberate and persistent demise of student support systems in this country' and was 'blind to the gross deficiencies of the scheme that he administers'. He argued that the value of income support to young people had diminished because the real value of allowances as well as access to them had been reduced. Allowances were no longer intended to 'maintain students fully but to contribute to the cost of their maintenance', and fewer students were entitled to the (means-tested) allowances because fewer parents met the income criteria. This had come about because the upper limits for parental incomes had not been increased with inflation, and thus parents had to be 'very much poorer' before their children qualified for allowances than was the case originally.

Dawkins claimed that between 1976 and 1979 these factors had caused the proportion of university students eligible for allowances under TEAS to fall from 40 to 35 per cent (p. 422). The primary aim of the original TEAS—to increase access to tertiary education—was therefore not being achieved. In the following year, 1982, during a parliamentary debate on schools funding, Dawkins referred to the other issue that was to become increasingly significant in the consideration of youth income support, namely school retention rates:

> There is a very clear need to concentrate . . . on the problems of school retention rates because we have found that retention rates, after 25 years of increasing gradually, in recent times have turned around. We now find that more and more kids, mainly boys, entirely those in government schools, have been dropping out of school much earlier than was the case a few years ago. (Hansard, HR, 1982: 970)

The immediate context for the policy development processes examined in this chapter was the policy speech delivered by Bob Hawke, then Leader of the Opposition, at the start of the ALP's campaign for the March 1983 election. Hawke gave a lot of attention in his speech to youth issues and identified three factors that should drive new policies in this area. He referred first to education, noting that when compared with the OECD countries, 'Australia has one of the lowest retention rates for later year school students'. He then referred to youth unemployment: 'Too many young, unskilled Australians are looking for jobs and by doing so are increasing the size of the workforce when insufficient jobs are available . . . The problem of youth unemployment in Australia is extremely serious and undoubtedly getting worse' (AFR, 17 February 1983: 10). Hawke went on to refer to national productivity, arguing that to compete in the world would require Australia to improve its educational and training standards.

STRUCTURES AND PLAYERS

The appointments and organisational arrangements that were made for the administration of youth affairs immediately after the Hawke Government's election in March 1983 were a crucial step in following through the priority given to youth affairs in Hawke's election rhetoric. In particular, the changes made in the location, role and resourcing of the **Office of Youth Affairs** (OYA) were of great significance for the development of policy on youth income support because they provided the impetus for the energetic study of issues and policy options over the next year or so.

Following the election, Senator Ryan became Minister for Education and Youth Affairs with Dr Peter Wilenski supporting her as Secretary of the Department. To strengthen the capacity of Ryan's new department to provide policy leadership in 1983, the OYA was transferred from the Department of Employment and Industrial Relations to the Department of Education, renamed the Department of Education and Youth Affairs. Its initial role was to improve coordination and consultation between federal, state and local governments on the handling of youth issues.

In May 1983 the department was given an explicit policy leadership role as convenor of an **IDC on Youth Policies**, with the function of coordinating all federal policies and programs affecting young people. This IDC was to be the main coordinating mechanism, its task to examine a comprehensive approach to youth policy, including youth allowances. More specifically, it was required to look at

- rationalising the structures and levels of income support for young people;
- relating education and training to changing social, economic and technological conditions; and
- enlarging and integrating the range of alternatives available to youth in education, training and employment (DEYA 1983a: 17).

The agencies represented on the IDC were the **Departments of Education and Youth Affairs**, **Employment and Industrial Relations**, **Social Security** (DSS), **Prime Minister and Cabinet** (PM&C), **Finance**, and **Treasury**. DSS was represented by the **Social Welfare Policy Secretariat** (SWPS), a think-tank within the Social Security portfolio. There had been a similarly composed IDC meeting on and off over the past ten years with little result.

The OYA was expanded and within a few months was upgraded to a division—at first with two and later with three branches and headed by Alan Abrahart until the end of 1984. A position of Special Adviser on Youth Allowances was created and filled in May 1983 to help the OYA provide policy advice to the government on rationalisation benefits and allowances for young people. That position was held by Meredith Edwards between May 1983 and August 1985. A new branch established in June 1983 was named the **Policy Development Branch** and given two main tasks: to assist a review of Australia's youth policies by an OECD team later in 1983; and to 'prepare options for the Government for a comprehensive approach

THE PLAYERS

Politicians

Coates, John	Backbench ALP Senator
Dawkins, John	Minister for Trade and Minister Assisting the Prime Minister on Youth Affairs, 1984–87
Grimes, Don	Minister for Social Security, 1983–84
Hawke, Bob	Prime Minister
Ryan, Senator Susan	Minister for Education and Youth Affairs, 1983–84 Minister for Education, 1984–87
Staples, Peter	Backbench ALP
Zakharov, Olive	Backbench ALP Senator

Public servants

Abrahart, Alan	Head, OYA (DEYA), 1983–84
Bowdler, Peter	Head, Student Assistance Division, DEYA
Cox, Jim	Policy analyst, SWPS
Dunlop, Marion	Senior officer, SWPS and seconded for three months to OYA
Dusseldorp, Jack	Head, OYA (PM&C), 1984–87
Edwards, Dr Meredith	Special Adviser on Youth Allowances, 1983–85
Halton, Charles	Chairman, Commonwealth Review of Youth Allowance Administration, 1985–86
Milligan, Bruce	Assistant Secretary, Student Assistance Policy Branch, DEYA
Moss, Don	Senior officer, DEYA
Phillips, David	Assistant to the Special Adviser on Youth Income Support, OYA
Podger, Andrew	Assistant Secretary, Social Welfare Branch, Department of Finance
Rogers, Vic	Policy Coordinator, SWPS
Rose, Alan	Deputy Secretary, PM&C
Stanton, David	Head, Development Division, DSS
Visbord, Ed	Deputy Secretary, PM&C
Ward, Ian	Assistant Secretary, Schools and Aboriginal Student Assistance Branch, DEYA
Wilenski, Dr Peter	Secretary, DEYA, 1983
Williams, Helen	Deputy Secretary, Department of Education, 1985–87, Secretary, DEYA, 1983–85

Other	
Freeland, John	Academic, University of Sydney
Garnaut, Ross	Senior adviser, Prime Minister's Office
Kirby, Peter	Chair, Committee of Inquiry into Labour Market Programs
Mawer, Allen	Senior Adviser to Minister Dawkins

to youth policies, particularly in the areas of education, employment, training and income support' (p. 17).

In 1985, when Dawkins took over responsibility for Youth Affairs, the OYA was moved to PM&C under Jack Dusseldorp. From that time, Allen Mawer as adviser to Minister Dawkins on youth issues and a little later, David Phillips, an officer assisting Meredith Edwards, became key players.

> *'If you gave Dawkins a responsibility, he would immediately look at ways in which the cards could all be thrown in the air and come down differently. That was just part of his temperament . . . No matter what job he was given, he would always be looking at a way, one, to make his name, and, two, shake up the world by challenging wisdom.' (Allen Mawer)*

IDENTIFYING THE ISSUES

In this section, 'identifying the issues' refers mainly, if somewhat arbitrarily, to certain activities undertaken from the election of the Hawke Government in March 1983, when a process and analytical framework were developed for converting the problems facing young people and outlined in Hawke's election speech, into operational programs consistent with his stated directions for change.

At the economic summit in April 1983 and beyond, the problem of youth unemployment was raised as an important issue facing the government. The new Minister for Education, Senator Susan Ryan, addressed the issue of the future of young people, given rising unemployment and the need for increasing their skills. There was widespread agreement at this point about there being too few young Australians remaining at school and continuing on to tertiary education, so the issue was not difficult to sell to the public. Later, some key trade-offs had to be faced by ministers—given the tight fiscal environment, how was the increase in educational participation to be financed?

'Nobody came to the table saying there is no problem. There was no one arguing for the status quo. Instead the argument was about what change [should occur].' (Allen Mawer)

One of the first actions of the Hawke Government was to invite the OECD to review and advise on existing programs and policies for young people. Thereafter the OECD contributed to policy-making in several ways. Most obviously, it provided an international perspective, something that does not always happen in policy-making, particularly if there is pressure to get results and limited time and resources.

The OECD review (1984) provided a focus for initial work by the Office of Youth Affairs because the latter was drawn into developing the review's terms of reference. Broad-ranging terms of reference were agreed which asked the review team to look at existing Australian policies and programs for people aged 15–24 years in the areas of 'education, training, employment and income support', and to suggest how the needs of such people could be better met. The terms of reference were preceded by a lengthy preamble, intended to convey the policy context for the review (pp. xxxii–xxxiv).

It was expected that the review would 'enlarge the Australian perspective of the complexity of the problems of young people and enable overseas experience of similar problems, and of approaches already tried elsewhere, to be taken into account' (DEYA 1983b: xxxii). Australia was not alone in its youth unemployment problems, and the government hoped that by inviting an OECD review of the situation it might benefit from the experience of other countries.

The review team was asked to comment on several specific matters, including 'the practicability of a comprehensive and integrated approach to support services for young people, as for example through a "youth guarantee", "youth allowance" or one of the various proposals of this kind developed overseas', and on the 'role of income support structures in providing incentives for young people to continue appropriate education and training' (p. xxxiii).

In its subsequent report towards the end of 1984, the OECD described the problem:

> Income support for young people is the single most controversial issue in the debate on youth policies in Australia. Though virtually everyone—government authorities, parents, young people and youth advocates—agrees that the current arrangements are in large measure complex, inconsistent and inequitable, and create perverse incentives, there is no consensus over how to make improvements. The 'gridlock' created by the present collection of arrangements means that every

proposed 'improvement' introduces a new complexity or inequity, reorders incentives, or is intolerably expensive; every proposed change makes new winners and losers. (OECD 1984: 56)

The second and significant way in which the OECD review stimulated the consideration of issues was through the background paper that the Department of Education and Youth Affairs, and in particular the OYA, was required to produce for the review, to help it 'focus quickly on the key issues' and to provide in one document comprehensive reference material on youth issues (DEYA 1983b: xiii). The paper, nearly 300 pages in length, was published later in 1983. It assembled a large amount of factual material on 'young people in the context of social and economic change', on trends in formal education and in the labour force experience of young people, and on the various employment and training programs of the Federal Government.

One of the more significant parts of the background paper, on the development of youth income support, was in the concluding chapter, 'Commonwealth Income Support: Programs and Issues'. Here four main issues were identified for attention: the complexity of the existing income support structure; equity considerations; incentive and disincentive effects; and dependency issues:

- *Complexity*. By 1983 there were over 30 different federal programs (and a further 30 state programs) under which young people could be given income support or other financial assistance, directly or through their parents.
- *Equity*. The allowances paid to young people differed according to the courses or institutions they attended or the activities they undertook, rather than to their social or economic circumstances; that is, young people in seemingly 'equal' economic circumstances and with similar 'needs' could receive quite different levels of allowances.
- *Incentives*. What effect do allowances and their different rates have on young people's attitudes towards joining the workforce or continuing their education?
- *Dependency*. At what point does a child become independent of his or her parents? This very complex social issue had a great bearing on each of the others, as it was necessarily implicit in judgments about what constituted equitable or 'effective' allowances or a 'perverse' system of allowances.

Preparation of the background paper was a key part of the issue identification stage, and it had a wider significance in the whole policy-making process as the main reference document. Its preparation was the catalyst for creating a small, albeit temporary, community of experts and analysts from within and beyond the bureaucracy, who would become involved to varying degrees over the next year or so in developing a policy for youth income support. This informal and loosely structured network of specialists could readily and informally discuss ideas and policy options with one another. Immediate responsibility for producing the background paper lay with staff in DEYA, in particular Alan Abrahart, head of the OYA. But staff from other agencies and universities contributed to drafting the paper and gave comments and advice on its contents. These included John Freeland, who was seconded for the exercise from the University of Sydney.

The other main event in 1983 that helped put youth issues on the agenda was the delivery of an address on youth income support in June 1983 by Peter Wilenski (1983: 1). The stated purpose of the address was to 'stimulate discussion and present information rather than advance a particular viewpoint'. Notwithstanding this disarming preamble, the paper presented a view of the issues, suggested principles 'that might guide the review and development of financial support structures [for young people] in the long term', and outlined possible models for these structures. Although it therefore addressed matters that, in the model of the policy cycle, 'belong' to a later phase of the cycle—including possible policy solutions—it was the type of scene-setting paper that is commonly delivered by a politician or senior bureaucrat at the start of a policy cycle, with the intention of taking the initiative.

After summarising the two main problems of youth unemployment and low school retention rates, in much the same way as these problems had been outlined in Hawke's election policy speech, Wilenski argued that the 'core of the youth unemployment problem' lay with those young people 'coming from a stratum of society whose life chances have *always* been poor' (p. 5), and that the priority in policy 'as a matter of both equity and efficiency should be given to the children of the twenty per cent of the population who are at the bottom of the socio-economic ladder' (p. 7). He noted failings in the existing system: inequities, 'perverse incentives between education and unemployment', and inconsistencies in approaches to income support and dependency of students on their parents. He suggested some principles (discussed below) that 'might guide the review and development for financial support structures in the long term'.

Identifying and articulating the problem in this case was not confined to the few months after Labor was elected in March 1983 but continued into 1985, the year major new reform directions were announced in the budget. John Dawkins, who took on the role of Minister Assisting the Prime Minister on Youth Affairs from January

1985 as well as Minister for Trade, played a key role in clarifying the problem and articulating it. For example, in a speech in Bathurst as late as July 1985, he set out the case for reform of youth income support arrangements. He referred particularly to Australia's need for an educated and skilled workforce if the country was to be competitive in the world economy. 'All too often, it seems to me the youth income support debate is conducted in a vacuum. As if it is an intellectual exercise which bears no relationship to the future capacity of Australia to earn its way in the world' (Dawkins, 7 July 1985: 8).

Partly because debate was still active within Cabinet on the nature of youth allowances, Dawkins was, in this speech, selling the need for education allowances to be at least as high as unemployment benefits 'to remove the present financial incentive for young people to leave education and training'; he used examples to make his point:

> Let's call our first example Christine. She's 16 and lives with her parents. They have trouble making ends meet. Christine has just finished Year 10 and has ambitions to get her HSC. When she examines her options she finds that the Government will pay her parents benefits totalling $28 a week for her to continue with secondary schooling. But should she leave school to look for a job, even if she fails to get one—which is one chance in five at her age—the Government will pay her $45 a week in unemployment benefits. Christine and her family would like her to continue in education but household income is their first priority so Christine leaves school. She finds that there are few jobs, and those that there are go to people who are older and/or have better qualifications than she does. She will find it extremely difficult to overcome that initial disadvantage in the labour market. (p. 8)

POLICY ANALYSIS

The boundary between 'identifying the issues' and 'policy analysis' can be difficult to define in practice. This is because the analysis can expose new problems or information that cause the original conceptualisation of the issues to be questioned, and those issues to be revisited. Identifying the issues can thus extend into subsequent phases of the policy framework, and as Wilenski's paper showed, policy analysis can also begin in the issue identification stage.

Here the policy analysis phase is defined as beginning late in 1983, when the OECD review team visited Australia and a meeting of federal and state ministers responsible for youth issues asked the Commonwealth to prepare a discussion paper on income support for young people. It also includes a period of intense deliberations by the Standing Committee on Youth Policies—an IDC of relevant officials—which developed principles and options for a comprehensive set of measures. The analysis phase is taken as ending about a year later, in December 1984, when Cabinet started to make decisions on the future of income support payments.

Policy analysis in this case, as with others in this book, can be usefully considered to have three key elements with some overlap in time: data-gathering and research; addressing key questions by decision-makers; and the clarification of objectives and developing of options. As will be seen, options were developed in some detail by the bureaucracy before they were seriously considered by ministers.

DATA AND RESEARCH

Between 1980 and 1983 a number of academics gave close attention to youth employment issues (e.g. Gregory and Duncan 1980; Gregory and Stricker 1981; Ironmonger 1983), and an important conference on these issues was held at the Australian National University in 1981. The report of this conference (Baird, Gregory and Gruen 1981) became a significant source of ideas for subsequent policy-making.

Many important research activities occurred during 1983–85, apart from the OECD background paper and the OECD Report itself:

- A major review of labour market programs, including youth programs (the Kirby Inquiry), which submitted its report to the government at the end of 1984.
- Bureau of Labour Market Research publications, including reports on youth employment issues in 1993. For example, its study 'Youth Wages, Employment and the Labour Force' (1983) concluded that employment of young people fell at the same time as their wages increased relative to those of adults. Debate ensued on the extent of this relationship.
- The OYA/SWPS document published early in 1984, *Income Support for Young People*, which identified at least 37 allowances young people could receive and put up for discussion a wide range of policy options.
- A paper researched and published by the OYA on evidence about the impact of educational allowances on incentives, *Education Participation and Financial Incentives* (OYA 1984). This was a response to the gap in knowledge about the extent to which financial factors influence a young person's participation in education. It found that 'marginal' groups of students were particularly susceptible to financial factors affecting participation

and were likely to be the students 'tipped out' by an unfavourable balance of financial and economic incentives.

- An ANOP survey of youth attitudes and opinions commissioned in November 1983. Its 1984 report, *Young Australians Today*, 'was designed to assist government in meeting the needs of young people and to help in communicating with them', 'The main message for government is that most young people have genuine fears and worries which are fundamental to their own identity. Most of this insecurity is employment related' (ANOP 1984: x).
- An Australian Bureau of Statistics (ABS) statistical profile of Australia's youth population, its main contribution to International Youth Year in 1985.
- Data arising from the Youth Affairs Council of Australia (YACA) consultations, which confirmed ANOP data. The findings of the YACA and ANOP studies 'have added to other data from a number of recent smaller, more specific or localised consultations, surveys and reviews on Australian young people, to provide a slowly emerging impression of what young people themselves think' (OYA 1985: 2).

Government was fortunate in this case that its key policy people were also research-minded: for example, Vic Rogers from the Social Welfare Policy Secretariat had worked for several years on broader income support issues.

Thus when Cabinet began to make key decisions on policies for youth income support, early in 1985, issues had been widely researched and discussed among those with an interest in the subject. Unfortunately, on a couple of particularly pertinent issues, like the impact of increased allowances on incentives to participate, while solid research was undertaken, the results were not conclusive.

KEY POLICY QUESTIONS

These are very difficult issues with either major cost implications or the potential to cause disadvantage for one group of young people in order to benefit another. Probably the hardest issue is what the relativities should be between educational allowances and UB. (Edwards 1985a: 3)

The IDC on Youth Policies met many times from May 1983 until the August Budget of the following year, setting some guiding principles for a comprehensive approach to youth policies and identifying and developing options in some detail. The committee put the income support options to one side to be considered after the release in February of the OYA/SWPS paper. It then developed policies to form the basis of some incremental changes to allowances in the August 1994 Budget.

> *'The age and circumstance under which an individual becomes independent of their parents was a key issue.' (Vic Rogers)*

The context in which policy analysis was undertaken was an extremely tough fiscal environment. The Labor Government was keen on major policy reforms at this stage, but only if they were consistent with the need to rein in the budget deficit, or at best involved minimal expenditure. Throughout the policy analysis phase, there was considerable tension between the Social Security Minister and his advisers wanting to protect the unemployed on the one hand, and the Education Minister and advisers wanting to provide incentives for education participation on the other, by effectively redistributing from the unemployed to those in education. It was on this basis that departmental officials fought out which department should get the limited resources to assist their client groups.

> *'The [bureaucratic] players acted to protect their clients and fought hard for resources on that basis.' (Alan Abrahart)*

Perhaps the most contentious issue was whether to place a family income test on 18–20-year-old unemployed people in order to finance higher education allowances for all young people.

One side of the argument was that higher education tends to be used by middle-income families or the well-to-do. Despite free tertiary education, the social and economic backgrounds of those at university had not changed significantly. Many argued that those with higher education earn significantly more over a lifetime. Why should the Australian taxpayer provide students with the same allowances as the unemployed, who were drawn mainly from lower income brackets? For some it seemed more logical to start reform of youth policies with additional education places than with increased allowances for students. (All these arguments were also canvassed in the HECS debate; see Chapter 4.)

The other side of the argument was, as Dawkins put it in his Bathurst speech in July 1985, that increasing payments for education up to the level of UB would provide more encouragement for young people to stay in education by removing the financial incentive to leave it.

Ultimately, fiscal constraint forced a debate about the appropriate way to handle the inevitable trade-off between providing greater incentives for young people to participate in education and protecting the adequacy of payments for the unemployed.

There were continuing uncertainties, which research was unable to resolve easily, around how important income support was as a factor in decisions to continue education or to seek work. The evidence seemed to be that increased allowances would increase participation in tertiary education, but there was no solid evidence to suggest that increased secondary allowances would make much difference to secondary participation rates.

DEVELOPING OBJECTIVES AND OPTIONS

While there was widespread agreement, inside and outside government, on the need for reform of income support arrangements for young people, different perspectives came to the fore when attempts were made to clarify the objectives of reform. The OECD report observed: 'The controversy over income support for young people seems to swirl around technical questions of how to "rationalise" the various arrangements without first fully recognising what purpose a rationalised income support system for young people might serve' (OECD 1984: 56, para. 2.22).

At the start of the reform process there was considerable lack of clarity about the purpose of existing secondary and tertiary allowances. TEAS, for example, was seen by some to be a top-up to parental support, quite distinct from the purpose of UB for a young person of the same age—parents were not expected to support their unemployed children. But reform of income support payments was being considered; people were increasingly regarding TEAS as an income support payment that could be compared with UB.

Minister Ryan weighed in and set out the government's intentions late in 1983:

> The government wishes to achieve a situation where by the end of this decade most young people complete the equivalent of a full secondary education either in school or in a TAFE institution, or in some combination of work and education. This objective is being pursued in the context of the overall view of youth policies being undertaken by the Government with the assistance of the OECD, aimed at providing young people with a range of options in education, training, employment and community activities and a more equitable and rational income support system to help sustain them in this period of their development. (Quoted in OYA/SWPS 1984: 34)

In its response to the OECD report, the government identified six objectives for future income support measures (DEYA 1985: para. 33):

- ensuring adequate levels of allowance
- a choice of options free of financial factors

- financial incentives to participate in post-compulsory education and training
- equitable treatment of the disadvantaged
- recognition of increasing maturity and independence
- the importance to society of education and training.

The Wilenski (1983: 15–16) models or options were based on a set of principles that contributed to determining what was to be achieved. They were progressively narrower in their coverage and less costly.

- Under his *General Model*, estimated to cost $2.8 billion a year, a youth allowance would be paid to all young people aged between 15 and 19 years who were not in full-time employment, 'to provide them with a financial base from which they can undergo further training or education' (p. 17).
- A *Modified Approach*, estimated to cost $1.5 billion a year, would provide all young people not in full-time employment with 'a basic allowance at a relatively low level', which, if supplemented with part-time earnings, would provide 'a basic minimum of support' (p. 19).
- A *Restricted Model*, estimated at $1.1 billion a year, would discard the idea of a basic universal allowance and focus on 'positive discrimination in favour of the needier individuals and groups' (p. 22).

The previous and subsequent history of youth income support policy in Australia could largely be written around shifts between the concepts implicit in these three models. Although a single and universal youth allowance was Wilenski's preferred position, it was not pursued further because it was too expensive. But his paper did provide an analytical framework for subsequent discussion on youth income support. It shows the power of a simple idea—a single youth allowance—that never lost its supporters and eventually came into existence at the beginning of 1999.

In January 1984, a few months after the DEYA background paper had been released, a discussion paper, *Income Support for Young People*, was produced jointly by the OYA and the SWPS. Its origins can be traced to a meeting of the State Youth Ministers Council in November 1983. Its purpose was 'to expand on [the background paper] and to indicate some of the major options to address' (OYA/SWPS 1984: 4). The paper was mainly the work of five people from the two organisations concerned: Alan Abrahart and Meredith Edwards from the OYA and Vic Rogers, Jim Cox and Marion Dunlop from the SWPS.

A WORDING EXERCISE

1 February 1984 Spent three hours arguing with SWPS (mainly Vic Rogers) over final wording for income support paper. Alan Abrahart also there.

3 February 1984 Meeting for two hours fighting over words and phrases with Vic Rogers of DSS and again from 3.30 p.m. to 5.30 p.m. Today was the day for getting paper together to deliver to Ministers . . . Had until 11 a.m. to make final amendments. Mad rush. A.A. just moved on to the next rushed job—consultation process once the paper is printed.

The paper put forward four principles for an improved system of youth income support: it should be simple; it should provide 'adequate' financial support for 'all young people in need'; it should be consistent with the broader aims of programs for young people, including participation in further education and training and attention to the needs of disadvantaged groups; and it should provide levels of income support sufficient to recognise aspirations for 'independence and self determination' among young people (p. 13). A concluding chapter presented four packages of options for changes to the existing income support arrangements. These were grouped according to the particular principles that were emphasised.

The first package emphasised consistency, especially between allowances under SAS (aimed at helping lower-income families support their children at school for Years 11 and 12), TEAS and UB. This package attempted in particular to address the question of consistency among incentives and disincentives for young people, as between education and seeking to enter the workforce. The second package gave more emphasis to the principle of simplicity, suggesting various forms of age-related education and training allowances. The third addressed the objectives of simplicity and consistency of the allowances structure with other educational and social security payments programs. The fourth gave more emphasis to the principle of adequacy in levels of income support, and thus recognition of young people's aspirations for independence; the single option in this package entailed increases in payments under the SAS, TEAS and UB programs.

The OYA/SWPS paper showed why systems of income support for young people have tended to be complex, and why much of the policy-making in this area has amounted to a search for simplicity. To address the four principles that it suggested should guide the determination of a youth allowance, it outlined sixteen 'illustrative' options and referred briefly to numerous other options that could also have been considered (p. 94).

The ongoing complexity of income support for young people stems from the fact that, as with many policy development exercises, such support is expected to meet several different and conflicting objectives. There is a tension between these objectives, the goal of simplicity, and the standing objective of efficiency that confronts all government programs.

> Here is a dilemma: to introduce a youth allowance which treats young people as financially independent of parents would cause a large transfer of resources from taxpayers to young people and in gross terms would be very costly; to introduce a single youth allowance by imposing a parental income test on Unemployment Benefit could be seen as transferring resources the other way. Further it would be more socially unacceptable, and would not assist in encouraging education participation particularly at a time when the range of economic activities available to young people is so restricted. (Edwards 1984: 110)

Simplicity can sometimes cost money, and this fact made development of a simple but equitable form of income support for young people a challenging task. The resolution of conflicts between equity and efficiency (including in this case economy in outlay and simplicity in administration) usually requires input from politicians, and the type of input necessary in this particular case did not come until early in 1985.

Producing a discussion paper of this kind with a wide range of options looked like an orderly step towards a solution, but in fact it was a reflection of the different perspectives and objectives of officials representing their agencies and therefore it was likely to be very difficult to develop a short list of options for Cabinet's consideration. If these options had been taken to Cabinet at this stage they could have led to confusion rather than set a direction for change; what Cabinet needed was to go back to basics and consider the key issues first. But the activity of the OYA, especially this discussion paper, was useful in generating community debate, and it appears to have had some influence over the decision in the 1984/85 Budget to reduce the differential between UB for young people and educational allowances (see below).

10 February 1984 Our paper is at last released. But on tenterhooks all day wondering whether it would be. Late afternoon, after several attempts to get to Minister's Assistant Private Secretary, we got the go-ahead—Minister assumed lack of Treasurer's response meant he was happy for report's release and that Grimes would interpret it that way. Similarly, Vic was disappointed he couldn't get his Minister to respond all day.

The PR people were absolutely superb. From a.m. they took over the dealings with the press and getting the mailing organised. Once we had the 'all go' at 4.45 p.m. they went straight to it and had finished by 5 p.m. Took copy to Helen Williams—A.A. had already done the same but she was kind enough not to let on. It is such a relief to have it out. Looks so good too. Meet the press Monday. Fitted in writing a background briefing for the press today.

3 March 1984 Yesterday I had a couple of hours at the airport before coming back [from Melbourne] and spoke with Ross Garnaut from the Prime Minister's Office. It was great to talk to Ross and he basically supported our proposal. He thought it would be a significant social reform if we got it through.

CONSULTATION

Consultation by both policy advisers and policy-makers with representatives of those potentially affected by policy changes can and usually does occur at all stages of the policy development process, both formally and informally.

By mid-1984 a considerable amount of analysis had been undertaken and published on the subject of youth income support. Some articles by academics and parts of official publications, already discussed, were highly technical and complex. Thus it was not surprising that the Department of Education noted in its 1984/85 Annual Report that after publication of the OYA/SWPS paper early in 1984, the OYA 'engaged in extensive consultation on possible ways of reforming youth income support arrangements' (Department of Education 1985: 41). This consultation occurred at several levels and in different arenas.

Consultation was extensive with stakeholders (such as YACA, Australian Union of Students, AVCC, ACOSS and state governments) as well as researchers. Interestingly, most organisations consulted were only lukewarm about the idea of a single youth allowance, at least in the shorter term; they were concerned about the priority needs of particularly disadvantaged groups of young people, which such a blanket measure could not take into account.

The Commonwealth provided funds to YACA and other youth bodies in 1983 to conduct nationwide consultation with young people to assist in informing government on the dimensions of the problem. For example, 'the need for money was widely discussed by young people in the YACA consultations and ANOP reported that the second main spontaneous issue raised by young people after employment/unemployment was "insufficient money and making ends meet"' (OYA 1985: 44).

YACA, while funded to be active in giving views to government on youth issues, was an organisation that promoted certain types of reform rather than analysing specific policy positions. Its focus tended to be on the needs of the young unemployed, and especially the homeless, rather than those who had the opportunity to access the higher education system, who were regarded as more privileged.

Consultation also occurred through public presentations. For example, Meredith Edwards presented a paper titled 'Youth Allowances—Issues and Options' at the 1984 Autumn Seminar of the ACT Division of the Royal Australian Institute of Public Administration, and shortly after this presented another, 'Youth Allowances: Incentive and Reform Issues', at the 54th ANZAAS Congress held in Canberra in May 1984 (Edwards 1985b). The former paper looked at some of the issues that had been raised in the OYA/SWPS publication on income support; the latter reviewed some of the studies of the relationship between education participation and financial incentives, and the implications of these for a single, universal youth allowance, free of parental income test. It concluded that such an allowance would be costly, would not protect the interests of disadvantaged groups, could be seen to discriminate against other people in need in other age groups, would be unlikely to have taxpayer support, and in fact could, as a guaranteed income, distort the choice of young people—more so than for other people—away from paid activity.

This section would not be complete without mentioning the role of Prime Minister Hawke in attempting to relate closely to young people. Before his 'Priority One' statement in August 1985, Hawke had a wide-ranging series of consultations and phone-ins with young people. He encouraged them to give him ideas to tackle their concerns. In his budget speech of August 1985, he said: 'Young people have made their concerns clear. Above all they are uncertain of their future, and they wish for the economic independence that comes from earning an income' (p. 3). He went on to say, 'so that the Government can continue to be aware of and understand the broad needs and concerns of young people, it will maintain and enhance mechanisms for consulting with young people . . . The Government, to mark the close of International Youth Year, will involve young people and their organisations in reviewing progress made with the strategy'.

MOVING TOWARDS DECISIONS

28 July 1984 [just before the 1984/85 Budget] The last week
has been (almost) unbelievable. In the afternoon we realised
we would have to come back to work at night since Budget
Cabinet had asked DSS to go away and revise its package of
measures. We went back at 8.30 p.m.—Alan Abrahart, Helen
Williams, Peter Bowdler and I. DSS informed us they were
going to produce five packages—each one we would need to
react to by working out relevant changes to TEAS and SAS
with our aim to reduce gaps between UB and those payments.
But DSS was very slow informing us of its packages.

At one stage around 9.30 p.m., DSS had a fire scare and
had to evacuate their building; about one hour later we heard
they were with their Minister checking out their proposed
packages. Throughout the night the packages came in slowly.
Alan finished writing a speech for the next day at 1 a.m. that
he had to give on behalf of the Minister next morning in
Goulburn. At that stage Peter chucked it in and Alan and I
took over the figuring. About 3 a.m. Helen said our TEAS
increases were too large given that we said we would only go
for marginal increases so as to only just close the gap. So Alan
and I had to recalculate all that Peter and I had done without
any basic data to help us. At 5 a.m. David Stanton from DSS
talked on the phone as I attempted to discover the indexation
factor to be applied to the single adult UB rate. 'Did you watch
the sunrise—it is very romantic . . . are you enjoying your first
year in government?'

H.W. insisted we calculate all figures precisely. While we
did, she neatly wrote out a screed that the Minister could
follow—5.45 a.m. we said goodbye to her—I presume she
remained and saw the typist at 8 a.m. Back home 6 a.m. . . .
I had about one hour's sleep. Kids up—off to school, maybe
another half-hour but I was anxious to tell Bruce Milligan I
may not make the SAS Evaluation Meeting. Just about to
shower and Ian Ward rings to say our figuring was wrong and
what numbers did we use? I got to work around 10.15 a.m.
and went to the SAS Evaluation Meeting—called out by Ian
Ward to discuss figures. I was only half there.

Lunchtime I decided to get some fresh air. 12.45 p.m. I
was just leaving my office when Warren Lang from the Minister's Office rang saying the Minister wanted her team at
Parliament House immediately. A.A. was in Goulburn; H.W., I

thought, was in bed (I rang her home but no answer). Ian W. was at lunch. Off I went. Minister was furious we weren't all hanging around and contactable—'don't they realise this is the most important day of the year?' Soon after she took me through Cabinet Budget decisions on DSS proposals, Ian Ward and Don Moss arrived; five minutes later Helen Williams. We all left after Minister explained the DSS position and that we were to work out a $40m package. Felt great that the Cabinet had allowed so much but as HW warned, that was not guaranteed. [A crisis] took up Cabinet time so our Minister did not have her proposals discussed by Cabinet.

19 August 1984 Alan and I were not involved at the very last stages of finalising Income Support budget measures. Apparently Cabinet made the decisions and H.W. and Student Assistance Branch provided the costs. A.A. was in Adelaide and I was in and out of the office all day. What has happened is a mockery of the whole process of review we have been involved in and one can't help being disillusioned. But I'm told that you can spend all your time as a public servant fighting to keep what you have.

THE EVENTS

The main restructuring of youth allowances and the introduction of AUSTUDY were announced in the 1985/86 Budget, but the August 1984 Budget started the process of reform. In that budget there were a number of changes to the system of educational allowances to ensure that more students would benefit from Commonwealth assistance. For example, living allowances under TEAS were significantly increased and the gap was reduced between the TEAS at-home rate and the UB for 16–17-year-olds leaving school. There was also a 15 per cent increase in the SAS allowances. UB was also increased, but by less than education allowances. In his budget speech the Treasurer announced that there was to be a fundamental review of youth income support arrangements in time for the 1985/86 Budget to be undertaken by the IDC on Youth Policies, building on the OYA/ SWPS discussion paper. This would enable the government to introduce new youth policies and programs in the 1985/86 Budget (Department of Education 1985: 41).

In the second half of 1984, consideration of youth income support was caught up in the wider consideration of employment problems as a result of the Kirby Inquiry, around which there was also extensive involvement of the youth sector and related consultations. This inquiry had been initiated by the Hawke Government in December 1983, with a broad charter to examine labour market policy and programs and recommend improvements. Although youth employment issues were just one part of the field covered by the inquiry, and had by this time been the subject of intensive study by officials and academics, the government was anxious to develop a comprehensive approach to employment issues.

The decisive phase in the development of a new policy for youth income support began immediately after the re-election of the Hawke Government in December 1984. In a ministerial reshuffle at this time, Dawkins became Minister Assisting the Prime Minister for Youth Affairs, in addition to his main responsibility as Minister for Trade. OYA was moved to PM&C, coinciding with the International Youth Year of 1995. Direct accountability of the OYA to Dawkins and the Prime Minister, and the upgrading of the director position, which was given to Jack Dusseldorp, a private sector person interested in youth issues, lifted the profile of the OYA further and clearly signalled the priority that the Prime Minister intended to give youth issues in the government's next budget. An article in the *AFR* (12 December 1984) picked up the significance of Dawkins' appointment and the organisational change that the Prime Minister had taken over responsibility for youth policy.

Policies are normally developed in line departments for their ministers, and are tested by Cabinet and the central agencies for their consistency with key policy directions (chiefly PM&C) and for their cost-effectiveness and fiscal impact (chiefly Finance and Treasury). Situating OYA in PM&C meant that policy development took place there, rather than the traditional role of critically appraising line department initiatives. All this looked good to the youth community in International Youth Year, but it remained to be seen what in fact could be delivered.

The main focus of OYA at this stage was on traineeships and other programs to help young people access services. Dawkins and his office were interested in developing traineeships as a central focus of the 1985/86 Budget. But Dawkins also had a strong interest in income support options, so much so that he saw this part of the package as a way he really could make a mark on social policy reform. An added window of opportunity was that 1985 was International Youth Year. Income support policies were developed outside the branch structure by Meredith Edwards, with one assistant, David Phillips.

Dawkins quickly invigorated the policy-making process once OYA moved to PM&C. The power of a determined and persuasive minister can be seen from this point on. Dawkins had benefited from having been the Minister for Finance and so knew 'how to do over Finance'. Even so, at one stage he almost gave up (see below).

A critical point was when Dawkins put a youth income support submission to Cabinet in January 1985 as the beginning of a process to obtain resolution on some key questions. He was taking advantage of renewed interest among his colleagues on employment issues after Kirby's submission of his wide-ranging report to the government late in 1984, and also receipt by the government at about that time of the OECD report on youth education and employment. At that meeting, with the use of graphs and charts he had painstakingly overseen, his aim was to educate his colleagues and convince them of the seriousness of the problem—'to show them what a mess the allowances were in'. Dawkins also judged that it would be best to have the presentation by officials as well as himself. Key questions for Cabinet consideration were presented, but only in the context of broad options.

He did not want decisions at this stage but he did want to influence the thinking of his ministerial colleagues before the imminent round of savings papers that they would be considering.

> **30 January 1985** Yesterday was the first substantive Cabinet meeting of the second Hawke Government. As a result I spent most of the long weekend as well as days before preparing for that with Alan Abrahart, my boss and Allen Mawer. The distinctive feature of this meeting was to be Dawkins' presentation on Kirby and the OECD report as well as on income support—both issues and broad options. Alan and I were lined up to assist Dawkins with the presentation but not knowing how much he or we would do until the last minute.
>
> On Monday (Australia Day) at 4 p.m. we saw Dawkins and showed him the charts we had prepared for the meeting, lugging them into Parliament House. We spent an hour and a half with him. He made minute changes to the charts, including the colour of lines we had used for TEAS, SAS and UB. I came away most impressed with his combined eye for detail and a strategic big-picture focus.
>
> The next day we went into the Cabinet Room and sat at the back. Prime Minister Hawke turned to Dawkins to ask what was to follow. Dawkins explained and gave an introduction using ANOP survey material. Then Alan spoke for around twenty minutes on traineeships, using some charts. He spoke very well. About halfway through Alan's talk, Dawkins spoke with Allen Mawer, and Allen said to me that Dawkins wanted me to to do the whole talk on income support. After I finished,

in time for questions, most of the questions were on income support issues, e.g. whether our IDC was concerned about the lack of education places, whether low-income families would be worse off than pensioner beneficiary families, whether the latter would be worse off if there were a new home as well as away-from-home rate for 18 year olds plus UB recipients, and whether it was really turning the clock back to treat young people as dependants of their parents.

The key questions arising in IDC meetings and other places on which Dawkins needed decisions included:

- What should be the relativities between the level of UB and educational allowances?
- How much should those living away from home receive compared to those living with their parents?
- What should happen to personal and parental income tests, e.g. should the unemployed be treated differently from students?
- How should special needs groups be treated, particularly young people from pensioner/beneficiary families?
- Given limited funds, how should rates of allowances be rationalised?
- What transitional arrangements should be made to protect losers?

These issues would be very difficult to resolve and had big cost implications. It was obvious that any debate would be especially intense in Cabinet on the issue of relativities, reflecting strong differences of view in the IDC and elsewhere (see below). There was also the question of what to do with the non-mainstream or more minor student allowances, but that could be shelved until in-principle decisions could be taken on how to rationalise the main payments of TEAS, SAS and UB. Because getting agreement from Dawkins' colleagues was difficult, compromise along the way was inevitable.

'There was a genuine interest within government for increasing education participation. There was also a genuine interest of government in poverty issues and they [Ministers] had a difficult trade-off to make and they were finding it very hard to do. As a result you tended to have the tensions played out through surrogates.' (Vic Rogers)

Cabinet asked officials for further work on options. Because of the complexity and the wide variations in costs of different options for income support, an exhaustive process followed to show the implications of various options, with many submissions and memoranda for Cabinet produced between January and April 1985. At this stage an IDC process was not used; instead Dawkins relied heavily on Allen Mawer in his office and Meredith Edwards in PM&C, with a few key officials from Finance, Education and Social Security also involved. In the light of earlier Cabinet consideration of important questions to be resolved, Dawkins reduced the large number of policy options that had been published in the OYA/SWPS paper to a much smaller number that could be presented to Cabinet and that met ministers' concerns. Dawkins' submissions normally went first to a Taskforce of Ministers on Youth Matters. The relevant Caucus subcommittees also scrutinised possible decisions several times. Dawkins needed to go through this process of many submissions to try to narrow areas of disagreement with his colleagues and so 'avoid the dopey savings options' that would otherwise have arisen from the Department of Finance.

In the first half of 1985 ministers had great difficulty coming to an agreement on a cost-effective package of measures. Not unexpectedly, the Department of Finance, and to a lesser extent the economics area of PM&C, were attempting to keep down costs by options that would result in placing a family income test on the young unemployed. But increasingly, as proposals for income support arrangements came forward that left losers among the unemployed to finance higher payments for students, the Labor Left—effectively through the Education Caucus subcommittee—became more involved; they were nervous about measures seen to disadvantage young unemployed in relation to students.

> *'Because the social security interests in Caucus were very strongly left wing and quite out of sympathy with most of what Cabinet was trying to do on the rationalist front, the government didn't spend too much time trying to persuade them. They were left talking amongst themselves while the main game got away from them. Caucus, quite unusually for a Labor government, was a marginal player.' (Allen Mawer)*

A Youth Policy Taskforce was also established within OYA, in April 1985, to prepare a major statement on youth issues to accompany presentation of the 1985/86 Budget. It was chaired by Jack Dusseldorp and included other staff from the OYA and representatives of Employment and Industrial Relations, Education, and Community Services and also academic consultants.

BUDGET MEASURES

The statement issued by the Prime Minister, Bob Hawke, for the August 1985 Budget, 'The Commonwealth Government's Strategy for Young People', foreshadowed a comprehensive package of measures in three main areas: job training, financial support and education (Hansard, HR, 20 August 1985: 67). In terms of youth income support, the Prime Minister announced:

- an increase from 1986 of around 20 per cent in effective rates of secondary and tertiary allowances as the first step but with an intermediate rate of benefit for 18–20-year-old unemployed people from November 1985
- from January 1988, a 'common basic rate of allowance for 16 and 17-year-olds whether unemployed or students'
- from January 1988, 'a common rate of allowance for the single unemployed aged 18–20 years and tertiary students aged 18 and over who live away from home or are independent'
- from January 1989, a 'common basic rate of allowance for both secondary and tertiary students aged 18 and over'
- from May 1986, 'entitlement to rent assistance for unemployed aged 18–24 who are in private rental accommodation'.

In announcing the AUSTUDY reforms, Dawkins and the then Minister for Finance, Senator Walsh, had this to say:

> Following a detailed review of the main schemes providing youth income support, the government has decided to introduce age-related rates of allowance for 16–20 year olds, which, after a phasing-in period will provide, subject to income test, similar basic benefits to people of the same age regardless of whether they are in secondary or tertiary education, or, in the case of 16 and 17 year olds, unemployed.

> The rationalisation of youth income support programs is an important part of the government's comprehensive youth strategy, which aims to ensure that young people entering the labour market are better prepared and have the skills and qualifications necessary for economic independence. (Dawkins and Walsh, 1985: 18)

This was a time of considerable budget pressure and there was little room for additional expenditures. Despite youth initiatives being the top-priority budget item, the package of measures reflected this budget constraint in two main ways: in the establishment of the less than popular intermediate rate of UB for 18–20-year-olds, and in the clever phasing in of the common youth allowance.

The phasing in of the changes not only enabled some cost savings but allowed more time to work out how other education and unemployment allowances, targeted to special groups, could be integrated with the common basic allowance now proposed, without inadvertently introducing new problems.

The subsequent youth package, announced in the 1986/87 Budget, placed its main emphasis on traineeships and income support, but broad-based strategies to improve on education, training and labour market measures were included. It also encompassed changes to non-mainstream income support programs (see next section).

It is worth noting that in the 1987/88 Budget, the part of the package Dawkins and the Department of Finance had originally favoured was brought into effect without too much fuss: a 'dramatic curtailment of junior UB and vastly accelerated movement to a common allowance' (Andrew Podger, letter to author, 1999).

DIARY OF A PLAYER

3 March 1985 On Thursday Caucus [committee] met to discuss what Dawkins wanted to put to Cabinet on income support. He informed them that their minutes from the previous meeting had been leaked and that Michelle Grattan would run the story in the *Age* (the story also appeared in the *SMH*). He was not amused. There was opposition to taking from the unemployed to redistribute to those in education. After the meeting the Minister asked me back to his office and we discussed how to modify the proposal in the light of those comments.

18 March 1985 Monday was the day of Dawkins' submission to Cabinet on his youth income support proposal. I was in his office with Allen Mawer from 10 a.m. when Cabinet started, as we had arranged, in case Dawkins needed any costings done. Had arranged a 'hotline' to Finance for that. At 1.30 p.m., when the Minister returned, Allen Mawer and I, with Dawkins' guidance, drafted a Cabinet Decision based on what ministers and note-takers believed to be the outcome. At that point Dawkins, while wording the draft decision cautiously, seemed to think Cabinet had agreed in principle to a 'common allowance', for 16–17-year-olds and convergence of rates for 18+ students and unemployed. Our draft was taken to the Minister in the Cabinet Room.

That afternoon or evening Cabinet . . . changed it so that no decisions were actually made but more consideration was to be given to the common allowance etc. This was Monday. On Wednesday p.m. I still had not seen the final decision. Monday night I thought we had really achieved something and couldn't sleep for excitement. But not having known what happened when Cabinet had a look at the draft that night, I was not correct.

On Wednesday it was more depressing when I saw the Ministers' alterations to the decision. There were not many but sufficient to make the decision not a decision at all except for more work. PM&C people say everything is now to be considered in the budget context and had talked of reconvening the wretched IDC . . . Dawkins has no intention of using an IDC.

2 April 1985 At work I have been depressed at lack of morale in OYA and lack of clear policy functions. We will lose the quality staff it has taken eighteen months or so to hire. Jack Dusseldorp's unavailability often means Alan Rose is our de facto head. Role of Economic and Social Policy Division—not giving me staff support but wanting to vet what I write to the Minister on income support. Stuck. I haven't been able to get much done because of lack of staff. I probably take all this far too seriously.

27 April 1985 Back after Easter and called to talk to the Minister. The first thing he says when I entered was 'We have to push this along faster than it has been going'. At that point we had planned on a Cabinet submission for ten days away. He had thought he would put it before ERC the following Monday (one week earlier than we had planned). He started to talk options, not having seen my paper with five options in it. I showed him the paper but he only read part of it . . . Allen Mawer pushed his favourite option (age-related by single year) and I pushed another (phasing in over two–three years) or combination of the two. Minister quizzed us on pros and cons and quickly discarded the type of PM&C option of phasing in over three + years and said he couldn't make up his mind on which of the [other] two options. He would let us know the next day . . . (he didn't).

Allen and I sat down for about an hour to summarise those two options to assist in his decision . . . On Monday I talked to Dawkins, who decided on Allen's option despite my strong advice to the contrary. That option aligned rates for 16–17-year-olds and 21+ year-olds but not for 18–19-year-olds, even when all phasing in had taken place. We wrote our draft Cabinet submission (for distribution Wednesday a.m. and comments by Thursday noon for lodgment Friday noon) when on Wednesday a.m. I heard from Allen that Dawkins had changed his mind and now supported my option. Changed draft submission quickly— was being typed in Dawkins' office anyway, partly because of lack of typing facilities in PM&C. This week I have had to use more than three different typists on three different floors . . .

David Phillips, so new to the job, having joined about ten days before Easter, could not have known what had hit him, although he coped really well.

Thursday Caucus [committee] met to hear from Dawkins what was to be in his submission. Another bombshell: Peter Staples and Olive Zakharov (of the Left) tabled 'Option 3' for Cabinet consideration. The next day and over the weekend I spent costing the Staples-Zakarov option, which was reported in the *Age* on Saturday morning.

This Monday morning was the day for Cabinet to consider the submission. Cabinet considered it for at least two hours. A taskforce of six ministers with well known different philosophical positions was to meet at 1 p.m. that day to resolve issues. Officials went to that meeting. They could not bring themselves to freeze UB for 18–20-year-olds. Dawkins was left to concentrate on the 16–17-year-old age group. He is obviously tiring of the issue. If Walsh won't spend any savings from youth and social security initiatives, there is no room for manoeuvre.

12 May 1985 A few weeks have passed since the Taskforce of Ministers met. By Thursday, 2 May, we had yet another draft submission out and back, and a document prepared on which the submission was based setting out a couple of options and stacks of variants. What a pace! Submission lodged Friday and to ERC on the 6th (Monday). Allen Mawer wrote the submission. I was despondent about its chances. Dawkins back from Korea on Sunday 5th and into the ERC the next morning. I saw submission Sunday night and decided on changes to it. Allen worked on document overnight and rang me early Monday to do the costings. When we eventually saw the ERC decision on Thursday (9th) it really gave Dawkins what he wanted—an in-principle decision along the lines of his proposal for an age-related youth allowance.

18 May 1985 Ministers met on Tuesday 14 May . . . Significant and expected differences of view emerged among ministers. A dismal occasion but at least it let officials off the hook for indecision. On Friday morning I was depressed because there was little more officials could do. It is now a matter for politicians, who are really very divided on where it all should go.

25 May 1985 Sunday 20 May, ministers met and reached some agreement as well as on issues yet to be resolved. Monday and Tuesday a.m. we drafted a submission for Monday 28 May meeting and did attachments Tuesday. Out to departments Wednesday. Wednesday afternoon held a meeting with departments on it. Thursday received coordination comments and sent the submission for printing. Horrid rushed day as changes to submission made as I heard from Halton and Rose, which meant I had to adjust costs apart from administrative arrangements. I was exhausted that evening and resigned to giving up. Arrived at work on Friday to hear our item had been taken off the Cabinet agenda by the Prime Minister. Thursday night three Caucus committees had met and resolved that there would be no parental income test (Dawkins was overseas this week). Apparently at Caucus committee meeting last night there was a phone call from a minister, who said to Chairman Coates, among other things, that the proposal was 'unworkable'. ANU Sociology has advertised for a senior research fellow. I think I should apply.

15 July 1985 Cabinet has decided effectively to defer further consideration of our proposals. Halton has been given the job (at my encouragement) of working out policy options in consultation with me. A Taskforce on Youth Policy has also been set up to write a Policy Statement for the PM. So I have been hopping between taskforces and trying to run a branch of people with low morale.

One exciting thing to happen (last weekend) was Dawkins' speech (in Bathurst) to a Youth Forum. I wrote the background paper to the speech, which linked the need for youth income support reform to the broader needs of the economy. I enjoyed that (done basically one morning at home). Halton saw it in draft and made a few comments, some of which AM accepted, but Dawkins speaking out caused quite a storm—breaking Cabinet solidarity—and Halton then said I should have given Dawkins a note on pros and cons of timing of that talk. It had never crossed my mind—just responded to a request for a background paper. One problem in the Public Service is that blame can be imputed to you but very little praise.

31 July 1985 Yesterday Cabinet decided on education and unemployment rates from 1986 to 1989. We think we have a major victory. Hung around Dawkins' office all day, occasionally responding to his requests for data. He unnerves me with his brightness and always being one step ahead. Spent the last two weekends on several submissions. In fairly high spirits until Sunday when Allen Mawer said . . . the Minister wanted $70 and not $73.30 per week for the TEAS living-away-from-home rate for 1986. So I sent Dawkins a strong brief, based on evidence, arguing against that and copied it also to the Prime Minister's office. Dawkins agreed to $73.30. The remaining problem is that the Prime Minister, Treasurer and Finance Minister are left to write the text and hence how the linkage is to be established in the future.

24 August 1985 We did have a major victory three weeks ago, and we had lunch for the 'workers' on income support across departments. To make sure Dawkins came I wrote a note to him inviting him to a 'Youth Income Support workers lunch'. He turned up and gave a very nice informal speech. I acknowledged the importance of his determination and single-mindedness. His next target is the education system, to make it more responsive to the needs of the economy.

The press followed these events closely. Front-page headlines in July and August conveyed well how the political argument evolved and Dawkins and the Prime Minister prevailed.

IMPLEMENTATION

The 1985/86 Budget provided a framework of decisions based on comprehensive analysis rather than detail. Hence there was a lot of clarification required on policy details through the implementation process yet to occur.

Two further steps were necessary to translate the principles outlined in the Prime Minister's August 1985 Strategy for Young People into workable programs. The first was to decide the details of the new structure of allowances to begin in 1988. These details, which were largely resolved by officials during the first half of 1986, were incorporated in the measures introduced in the 1986/87 Budget under the general program title of 'Priority One: Strategy for Young People' (Dawkins 1996).

Determining the details of the measures that were to be announced in this budget involved lengthy discussion between officials from the Department of Education in Canberra, in particular David Phillips and those officials in state offices who would be responsible for administering the new arrangements. It was fortunate that Phillips, who had worked in OYA in PM&C at the policy development stage, was now in the Department of Education and provided needed continuity between policy and implementation. He belonged to an implementation team that worked directly to the division head.

State officials were involved through several position papers issued

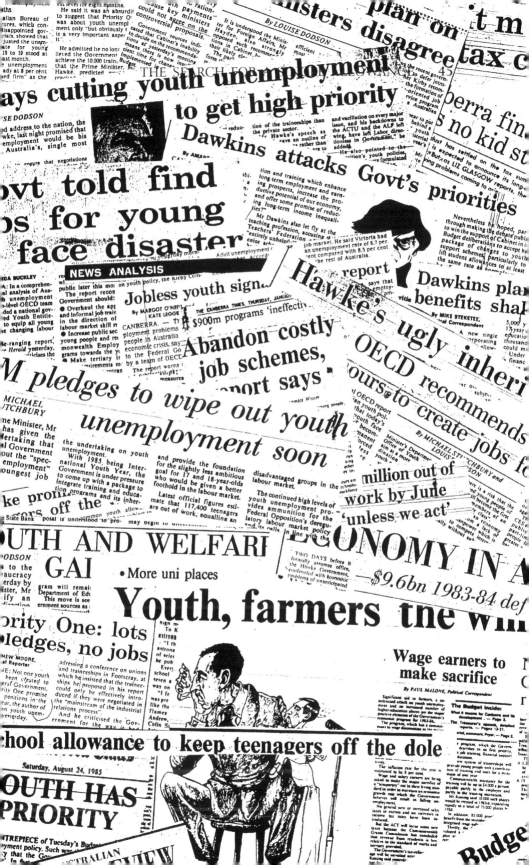

THE SEARCH FOR ...

ays cutting youth unemployment to get high priority

By LOUISE DODSON

Dawkins attacks Govt's priorities

ovt told find obs for young face disaster

Hawke's ugly inheri...

Dawkins pla... benefits shal...

By MIKE STEKETEE

NEWS ANALYSIS

Jobless youth signa...

By MARGOT O'NEIL KATE LEGGE

$900m programs 'ineffecti...

Abandon costly job schemes, ...port says

OECD recommends ...ours to create jobs fo...

By MICHAEL ST... ...CHBURY and LOUIS...

M pledges to wipe out youth unemployment soon

By MICHAEL ...UTCHBURY

... million out of work by June 'unless we act'

...ONOMY IN A... — $9.6bn 1983-84 def...

UTH AND WELFAR... GAI...

By ...ODSON

• More uni places

Youth, farmers the wil...

...rity One: lots ...ledges, no jobs

By ...EW MOORE

Wage earners to make sacrifice

By PAUL MALONE, Political Correspondent

...hool allowance to keep teenagers off the dole

Saturday, August 24, 1985

...OUTH HAS PRIORITY

The press

Judging from articles in the main Australian newspapers, the press focused largely on reporting episodes in the development of policies on youth income support, and provided comparatively little editorial or other comment on events. It was mainly interested initially in reporting the youth unemployment problem that provided the context for reviewing income support for young people.

For example, in December 1984, the report of the OECD team on youth unemployment was extensively covered: 'OECD recommends reducing hours to create jobs for young' (Michael Stutchbury and Louise Dodson, *Australian Financial Review*, 14 December 1984: 4); 'Jobless youth signal crisis: [OECD] report' (Margot O'Neil and Kate Legge, *Age*, 14 December 1984: 5); and 'Government told to find jobs for young or face disaster' (Amanda Buckley, *Sydney Morning Herald*, 14 December 1984: 3).

There was also one article about the same time that picked up the organisational changes that had great significance for the development of youth income support. An article by Louise Dodson in the *Australian Financial Review* on 12 December 1984, under the heading 'Youth and welfare gain in shuffle' (p. 3), noted that 'The Prime Minister has taken over responsibility for youth policy, which was previously part of Senator Susan Ryan's Education & Youth Affairs portfolio . . . It will now be the central co-ordinating body for youth policy and have an input into the development of all government programs which are thought to affect youth.' The article also picked up a change that had even greater significance for youth income support policy—namely the appointment of Dawkins, the new Minister for Trade, to also assist the Prime Minister in Youth Affairs.

During 1985, the press particularly focused on the initiatives being taken by Dawkins (discussed elsewhere in this chapter) and the political arguments stimulated by these initiatives. In March, Mike Steketee reported on a 'package of proposals' presented to ALP Caucus committees, involving 'a new single youth allowance' ('Dawkins plans benefits shake-up', *Sydney Morning Herald*, 1 March 1985: 1). In June, Louise Dodson reported that 'Federal Cabinet effectively shelved plans to rationalise youth payments because key ministers could not agree on the controversial proposals' (*Australian Financial*

Review), 4 June 1985: 7). The sequence of headlines during July and August convey well how the political argument evolved and Dawkins and the Prime Minister prevailed: 'Dawkins attacks Government's priorities on youth' (Amanda Buckley, *Sydney Morning Herald*, 8 July 1985: 1); 'PM pledges to wipe out youth unemployment soon' (Michael Stutchbury, *Australian Financial Review*, 15 July 1985: 3); 'School allowance to keep teenagers off the dole' (Paul Malone, *Canberra Times*, 31 July 1985: 1); and finally, 'Youth wins Budget priority' (Keith Scott, *Canberra Times*, 21 August 1985: 1).

by central office on each key issue that required change, and state officers in particular were involved in drafting instructions. However, the development of those instructions and the new regulations had to be accompanied by training of the officials who would be administering the new arrangements. There were difficulties in that process, for in the brief space of six months there was a need to ensure that the intentions of the Cabinet decisions were understood by all involved in implementation. Many had been in the department a long time; they were not involved in the policy development and had different views about the purpose of educational allowances.

Phillips had the task of translating broad Cabinet decisions into regulations that were specific and yet flexible, to allow some discretion for dealing with the many different situations of those who would be seeking income support. Phillips and his colleagues took advantage of this process to clean up what was a complex set of regulations and to get greater consistency, for example, in academic progress rules that differed across programs.

Second, the proposals before Cabinet in the first half of 1985 were primarily concerned with the major payments and their rationalisation. But there were over 30 other payments to young people remaining. Each of them needed to be looked at to see if they could be amalgamated with any resulting payment structure and whether service delivery could be simplified. Earlier in 1985 Dawkins had set up a Task Force on Youth Allowance Administration (TFYAA) under the chair of Charles Halton to examine ways of rationalising non-mainstream allowances and improving on the delivery of main allowances.

The chief objective of the TFYAA, from the August 1985 Budget on, was to recommend how various forms of youth income support to special groups could be incorporated into the general youth allowance. There were six distinct schemes targeted at particular groups: the Aboriginal Secondary Assistance Scheme; Aboriginal Study Assistance Scheme; Adult Migrant Education Program (Living Allowance and Living Allowance for Advanced English Courses in Technical and Further Education Institutions); Assistance for Isolated Children; Maintenance Allowance for Refugee Minors; and Soldiers' Children Education Scheme.

After intensive work by a very large group of officials up to March 1986 (a committee described by one of its officials as 'running by exhaustion'), the Halton Taskforce recommended retention of the six schemes, with rationalisations in administration reflecting the principles that Cabinet had endorsed early in 1985 for the new system of youth income support. The taskforce believed that their recommendations would lead to 'a comprehensive and coherent package . . . and a more integrated system of youth income support' (TFYAA 1986). Resulting changes were announced in the 1986/87 Budget. Consistent with the treatment of more detailed policy issues in other cases, it was difficult to get Cabinet's interest once they had agreed on AUSTUDY as a direction for reform; other problems were seen as the province of officials to solve.

> *'I remember feeling very strongly in Dawkins' office at the end of the process that there was not going to be a leap in the dark— there weren't going to be unintended consequences. We knew what the political downstream effects were going to be. And in fact that was the way it panned out for the most part. There were few surprises in the implementation phase.' (Allen Mawer)*

EVALUATION

Over time, administrative details of many policies, if not some of their underlying objectives, are often amended, typically but not only in a budget context. A policy that is evaluated after a few years in operation is therefore unlikely to be identical with the policy that was first implemented. This was certainly the case with AUSTUDY. Criteria for determining who should be eligible for assistance, the levels of allowances paid and the methods of paying those allowances were details central to AUSTUDY, and these changed substantially over its life.

> Income support programs have changed almost annually, in terms of one detail or another. Since different eligibility criteria, levels, and methods of payment, to take but three issues, all affect the uses to which schemes can be put, changes in all these serve to influence the objectives of the scheme. [A] tendency to post-hoc rationalisation has

dominated the history of student income support. It means that any analysis must take into account the fact that the objectives at one point in the history of a scheme may be entirely different, even inconsistent with those at another point. (Chapman 1992: 43–4)

Several evaluations were undertaken of AUSTUDY, both 'inside' and 'outside' the bureaucracy, including parliamentary reports.

Parliamentary committee reports in 1989 and 1991

In 1989, three years after AUSTUDY had been introduced, the House of Representatives Standing Committee on Employment, Education and Training examined one of the issues that had been behind the establishment of AUSTUDY, namely Year 12 retention rates (HRSC on Employment, Education and Training 1989). The committee was asked to inquire into 'the factors affecting student participation in post-compulsory education and training, including . . . the effect of student financial assistance schemes in encouraging students to stay at school and enter further education in the post-compulsory years' (p. xi).

The department argued in its submission to the inquiry that AUSTUDY and related forms of income support for young people had been 'a significant factor in the recent improvement in retention rates' (p. 21). The committee seemed inclined to accept this, concluding somewhat cautiously that such assistance was 'greatly valued by recipients' and 'helps to remove some of the barriers to participation experienced by low income earners'. It recommended that the financial assistance schemes be 'maintained or improved' (p. 27).

Two years later, in 1991, the same parliamentary committee reported on a wider-ranging inquiry into 'the provision, administration and effectiveness of student financial assistance schemes, with particular reference to the findings of the Auditor-General's report on the administration of the AUSTUDY program'. The Auditor-General, as part of his standing function of reviewing the efficiency of administrative procedures in government agencies, had investigated the processing of applications for AUSTUDY, its measures for controlling benefits, and its management of staff and computing services. This investigation found weaknesses in the processing of AUSTUDY applications, including long delays, and overpayments. In May 1990, not long after the Auditor-General had released his report, the Minister asked the House of Representatives Committee to review AUSTUDY, with the broad terms of reference quoted above.

The sequence of events just described illustrates a process that can often initiate and drive the evaluation of public policies. The process, which could be summarised simply as 'one question leads to another', begins with the exposure of administrative weaknesses through routine 'audit' processes and then extends in scope when these weaknesses seem to point to wider, systemic problems. In this case, the Auditor-General was a key agent in the evaluation of AUSTUDY, but other administrative review agencies or the media can also be important in initiating evaluations.

The 1991 inquiry of the Employment, Education and Training Committee, like many such inquiries, received many submissions from the public. This time the committee was more critical of AUSTUDY than it had been in 1989. It noted that AUSTUDY and two related programs (ABSTUDY and the Assistance for Isolated Children Scheme) had never been 'properly evaluated', and found it 'disturbing that billions of dollars have been spent on programs for which success or otherwise has never been assessed' (p. vii). It tried to address the basic question of whether AUSTUDY had been effective in achieving the government's aims. But its conclusions reflected the problems and frustrations that frequently arise when attempts are made to assess the effects of particular policies in the complex world of government.

> The Department of Employment, Education & Training provided information which shows clearly that retention, completion and partic- ipation rates in post-compulsory education have increased, but was unable to quantify the influence which AUSTUDY has had on these trends. Indeed, what data does exist suggests that AUSTUDY plays little role in influencing peoples' decisions relating to education.

> The National Union of Students stated that one of the basic prob- lems in any historical overview of Commonwealth support to students was that there has never really been a comprehensive state- ment by the Commonwealth as to what the policy intentions were for either TEAS or AUSTUDY. (p. vii)

The Chapman Report

This was undertaken by an ANU economist, Bruce Chapman, who was independent of the department but was asked to produce an options paper and given wide terms of reference. He was to address 'the appropriateness of the objectives of student assistance support (alternative objectives may be canvassed)' and 'advantages and disadvantages of the current scheme and alternative or modified schemes . . .' (Chapman 1992: 3).

The Chapman Report became an authoritative framework and source of reference for the ongoing development of policy on income support for students, essentially because it focused on key ques- tions ('why does student income support exist?', 'how effective has

AUSTUDY been?', 'in what ways could AUSTUDY be made more effective?'); it was analytically rigorous and comprehensive; and it involved extensive consultation with interested individuals and organisations, on a similar scale to that of the 1991 parliamentary inquiry. It was inconclusive, like that inquiry, about the effectiveness of AUSTUDY. In terms of its effects on young people's attitudes to education: 'one conclusion stands out; the range of factors which impact upon participation in post-compulsory education is far wider than those on which AUSTUDY is targeted' (p. 110). But it showed that the core issue for policy was related to targeting: 'The essential challenge for reform is to improve the targeting so as to ensure that the right amount of assistance is delivered to those who most need it' (p. viii).

The report also demonstrated how ideas can be transmitted from one policy process to another, through the personalities involved. Chapman had been a key adviser in the development of HECS (see Chapter 4), and one of the policy options suggested in his report on AUSTUDY was 'to allow prospective AUSTUDY recipients to increase their level of financial support if they chose'. It was suggested that this could be done through 'loans of a particular type . . . modelled on the current arrangements for the Higher Education Contribution Scheme' (p. x), and this idea was subsequently developed into the Supplement Loan Scheme now associated with AUSTUDY.

Parliamentary committee report in 1995

The 1995 inquiry into AUSTUDY by the Senate's Employment, Education and Training References Committee was, like the 1991 inquiry of the corresponding House of Representatives Committee, prompted by a critical report from one of the Commonwealth's administrative review agencies. This time it was the Commonwealth Ombudsman, who in his 1993/94 report had highlighted 'the persistence of several difficulties with the AUSTUDY scheme and its administration', including delays and errors in processing applications and inconsistencies between DEET and DSS with respect to eligibilities for income support (p. 1).

The terms of reference for the Senate Committee's inquiry focused almost entirely on the administrative problems with AUSTUDY that had been exposed by the Ombudsman and others, and the 24 recommendations in the committee's report were directed at improving the scheme's administrative details. The committee considered that the principal issues in its inquiry related to eligibility criteria for, and consistency between, AUSTUDY and other income support arrangements through DSS; student debt and debt recovery procedures; and the quality of advice given to AUSTUDY applicants. It noted that 'the apparent levels of dissatisfaction with AUSTUDY seemed not to be diminishing', and it referred to a recent research report by two Monash University academics suggesting that there had been some rorting of AUSTUDY by relatively wealthy families who had 'arranged their income and assets so that their children might be deemed eligible for AUSTUDY support' (p. 1).

While the Senate Committee's report might thus be regarded as an evaluation of 'administration' rather than 'policy', when it is related to the series of AUSTUDY evaluations that preceded it, it implicitly demonstrates how a 'policy' can be inextricably linked with its 'administration', and how over time evaluation of the one interacts with evaluation of the other.

Parliamentary committee reports such as those involved in evaluating AUSTUDY can be significant not only because they are institutionally separate from and independent of the executive arm of government, where policies are largely developed, but also because they typically reflect a wider range of political and public opinion than would normally be recognised in a particular policy process. In addition, they are a permanent feature of the institutional environment and so have a capacity for ongoing evaluation of particular policies.

CONCLUSIONS

> How many of us who sat around this table last year considered that there was a chance of getting income support provision for unsupported young people, let alone educational allowances up to the level of unemployment benefit, or a commitment to the indexation of education allowances? (Edwards 1986: 204)

There were many factors that could have stalled the process of reforming youth allowances in this period from 1983 until the end of 1985. This was a time when fiscal constraints were paramount, to the point that 'no cost' options were often called for. In addition, ministers and Caucus were nervous about measures that might be seen to either disadvantage unemployed young people, compared with students, and/or cause people to become losers. On the whole, bureaucrats and ministers were not convinced by the evidence that the proposed changes would significantly affect educational participation rates. Some senior bureaucrats, if not ministers, considered it more logical to begin reform of youth policies with additional educational places rather than increased support for students. But it was International Youth Year and other forces were at work.

One of the key attributes of this case that worked towards success in achieving policy outcomes was the heavy reliance placed on a comprehensive process of research and policy analysis. At the outset, problems of youth unemployment and low school retention rates were clear. But further clarification through research was needed to help pursue an appropriate direction for reform.

Ideally, key policy questions that ministers are likely to disagree on are teased out early in the policy analysis stage of the reform process. This allows ministers to clarify their objectives and send the right signals to bureaucrats about the purpose and principles of reform. This case is a good example of options being developed *before* ministers had that opportunity for real debate on contentious issues. Hence while options were developed by bureaucrats throughout 1984, and many key policy questions were hotly debated inside and outside government over this time, it was not until 1985 that Cabinet devoted time to debating key questions and provided some useful directions for bureaucrats.

Once ministers became closely involved, they were engaged for many months before reaching their decisions. The IDC process was replaced by their deliberations, which were based on many submissions tailored to ministers' concerns. As with other cases in this book, the limitations of IDCs can be seen when they operate from relatively narrow departmental perspectives, even if they reflect ministerial differences.

> 'Line departments wanted to protect their patch—policies, programs, staff and administrative capital—from the possible implications of policy, and subsequent administrative integration . . . The effects of departmental self-interest and attempts at boundary maintenance were more to delay the pace of policy change than to frustrate it completely.' (Bruce Milligan, letter to author, 1999)

The simple concept of a 'single youth allowance' and later a 'common youth allowance' was able to help the community identify easily with the proposed solution. Early in the piece, however, the researchers and analysts were fairly clear that this could not be achieved in one leap, and indeed history shows that it needed a decade for achievement, with determined protagonists pushing at every step. This case presents only part of that process, with AUSTUDY itself being phased in over three years.

> 'One of the lessons here is the importance of timing, including taking opportunities such as a fiscal crisis to cut through bureaucratic differences and compromises. The politically possible can

suddenly be greatly expanded. The art for the policy adviser is to recognise the opportunity, and to draw on all the previous research and policy analysis to develop more radical policy options that might previously have seemed too difficult.' (Andrew Podger, letter to author, 1999)

Although fairly common in government policy processes now, at the time the amount of collaboration across departments to achieve a fairly major structural reform was unusual. Until this point, youth policy changes, at least, were somewhat incremental and ad hoc, rather than systemically introduced, as in this case. In part the process towards reform was helped by having the OYA operate out of PM&C. It is arguable whether such reform could have been achieved by a line department at the time, regardless of the strength and determination shown by a minister such as John Dawkins.

Interesting issues arise in this case about the boundary between the role of the public servant policy adviser and that of ministerial policy adviser. A close relationship developed between Dawkins' adviser, Allen Mawer, and the Special Adviser on Youth Affairs, Meredith Edwards, and her assistant David Phillips, and some officials were somewhat critical of the apparent advocacy role played by OYA through these people as well as the close involvement of Mawer in writing Cabinet submissions. But those people saw their respective roles as clear and distinct and would not have seen this as a problem. More of a problem was keeping on side all the relevant players, including those in PM&C who tended to side with the Department of Finance in minimising any increase in outlays.

> ***27 April 1985*** There were comments yesterday from Ed Visbord at lunch on my return to the Office: 'Don't forget which Minister you are really working for. When the chips are down . . .' In other words do not fall in too close behind Dawkins on income support because that's a dangerous position to take!

The reforms that were achieved resolved very complex issues. In a time of fiscal constraint there were bound to be losers as well as winners. Reform of a more incremental kind could easily have resulted if the government had not been so sensitive to the youth vote and the lack of other substantive measures to place in a package of measures to be announced as part of 'Priority One' in International Youth Year. Thus an element of political opportunism can be detected here. As well as that, there was the clever concept of phasing the proposals in over several years and placing that process in legislation, an unusual move for the time.

The story of how and why AUSTUDY was introduced has been

told here, more or less chronologically. But above all, this case, like others presented in this book, shows how different phases in the policy framework overlap. Putting the problem on the agenda and articulating it to the point where action was possible took place over two years and could still be seen in the speeches of Dawkins a month before major in-principle decisions for reform were taken.

CHILD SUPPORT
CHRONOLOGY OF EVENTS FEBRUARY 1984 TO AUGUST 1989

1984
February Publication of an AGs report on a maintenance agency.

November Presentation of child support paper by Harrison et al. to Family Law Conference.

1985
June FLC establishes a subcommittee to consider child support options; government commissioned IDC on maintenance options.

July Letter from Justice Fogarty of FLC to AG on possible child maintenance reforms.

December Cabinet establishes a Ministerial Subcommittee on Maintenance; and FLC reports to AG recommending a formula-based administrative approach.

1986
February First meeting of Cabinet Subcommittee on Maintenance; SJS ANU Conference on Child Maintenance.

March Meeting of Cabinet Subcommittee on Maintenance to discuss terms of reference and priority issues.

May Cabinet agreed general policy directions on child support.

June Subcommittee on Maintenance finalised decisions and final report.

July Final report of Cabinet Subcommittee on Maintenance to Cabinet.

August Government announces intention to establish CSA and reform existing child maintenance arrangements.

October Tabling and publication of Child Support Issues Paper and consultations commence.

1987
January Important *AFR* article questioning the scheme.

March Announcement of introduction of CSS in two stages.

May CSCG established to advise on formula for assessment of child maintenance.

December Minister for Social Security introduces legislation into HR setting up CSA.

1988
May Consultative Group report *Child Support: Formula for Australia* tabled.

June Stage 1 introduced and CSA established.

August Budget introduces Stage 2 and *Child Support Act 1988* and *Social Security Act* passed.

1989
August CSCG reports on evaluation of Stage 1.

Three

From child maintenance to child support: An unlikely policy reform

Australia possesses a world-leading Child Support Scheme, which provides both financial benefit to the children of separated parents and revenue for government. It is based on a formula that determines, in relation to income, what non-custodial parents (NCPs) should pay for their children's support. In most cases, this is assessed administratively rather than by a court decision. The tax system is used to collect payments with deductions made from income.

The Child Support Scheme was introduced in two stages. Three main components of reform were introduced under Stage 1, commencing on 1 June 1988:

- the courts to assess amounts of maintenance the non-custodial parent is to pay, with the financial needs of children given a higher priority than all but essential commitments of parents
- a Child Support Agency (CSA) to collect maintenance payments from non-custodial parents covered by the scheme, through deductions from wages and salaries or by direct monthly payments
- the Department of Social Security to distribute payments to custodial parents, through monthly payments.

Stage 2, starting from 1 October 1989, varied the assessment procedure of Stage 1 by substituting administrative for court assessment of payments by the CSA with the application of a formula related to the income of non-custodial parents.

This chapter is about the role of policy processes in the development and implementation of this radical social policy reform. What follows concentrates on policy development of the first two stage of the scheme over the years 1985–87 and the subsequent implementation and evaluation of Stage 1.

HISTORY AND CONTEXT

From the mid-1970s, much attention in Australia focused on the poverty of most sole-parent families. Although the Family Law Act of 1975 specified that both parents had a financial responsibility to maintain their children according to their means, child maintenance was until the 1980s essentially voluntary; this was reflected in the proportion of sole parents who received regular maintenance payments for their children—less than 30 per cent in the early 1980s.

When maintenance payments were made they were usually quite low, averaging between $20 and $25 a week, on average only 13 per cent of take-home pay, with a 'going rate' being applied by the courts. There was almost no regard to the NCP's ability to pay—the higher the NCP's income, the lower the proportion paid in maintenance (Edwards et al. 1985) so one of the reasons for the poverty of sole parents was found to be the lack of financial support from NCPs. The child support reform process was therefore driven partly by a concern for equity.

No policy reform process, however, can be considered outside its policy and political context. In this case the child support reforms need to be looked at alongside the following external environmental factors operating in 1985/86 when the child-support issue was put on the agenda:

- a government needing savings (including reducing sole-parent pension outlays)
- increased recognition of the need to provide better financial support for lower-income families, especially sole-parent families, given their relative poverty
- the need for a more active labour market policy that would minimise disincentives to work
- a government keen to make its mark in moulding public attitudes towards quality family life.

In addition, a major review of social security began in 1986 (the Cass Review). One of its main recommendations, to increase financial support for families, needed a mechanism for financing, and revenue was expected for this purpose from reform of child maintenance arrangements.

An important attempt at child maintenance reform was started in March 1983 when the then Commonwealth Attorney-General, Senator Gareth Evans, set up a departmental inquiry, the National Maintenance Inquiry, to examine and report on maintenance systems and the possible establishment of a national maintenance agency 'to improve significantly maintenance enforcement and collection within Australia' (Attorney-General's Department 1984). The Report of the National Maintenance Inquiry, released in February 1984, presented clearly the inadequacies of the existing collection and enforcement system. It was less clear on how to solve the problem of inadequate maintenance payments, and it failed to relate the collection and enforcement of maintenance to broader issues of child support, since its terms of reference did not require it to do so. A number of organisations were therefore very critical of the report (Edwards 1986a; Holub 1989).

Since no existing department or agency was prepared to undertake the collection and enforcement of maintenance, and interdepartmental cooperation could not be counted on, the report advocated that a separate agency be established, at additional cost. Partly because of this proposal, the report was not able to show conclusively that there would be net savings in government outlays on sole-parent payments. The government saw this lack of clear budgetary savings as a weakness, and was also concerned at the administrative complexity of setting up an entirely new national agency (CSEAG 1992: 44). In addition, by the time the government considered the report, it realised the importance of changing the way payments were assessed, as well as improving the collection and enforcement procedure, if it were to gain significant savings.

This attempt at reform stalled mainly because of inadequate definition of the problem and lack of clarity about what the new agency was expected to achieve. Even if the initiative had led to government savings, it is arguable whether a savings option on its own, without broader social benefits, would have succeeded in gaining the support of most ministers, let alone the public. The reform agenda was picked up again by the government in 1985, initially in a search for revenue but also because of the increasing poverty of sole parents. How this story unfolds is elaborated on after the structures and their players are introduced.

STRUCTURES AND PLAYERS

From the second half of 1985 until he left his social security portfolio early in 1990, Brian Howe, as Minister of Social Security, was the main driver of the child support reforms.

Because several Cabinet submissions from a 1985 IDC on maintenance failed to produce any outcome, Howe had no difficulty in getting the Prime Minister's agreement to establish a **Cabinet Subcommittee on Maintenance**. This subcommittee consisted of Brian Howe (chair); Paul Keating, Treasurer; Peter Walsh, Minister for Finance; Lionel Bowen, Attorney-General; Susan Ryan, Minister Assisting the Prime Minister on the Status of Women; and Don Grimes, Minister for Community Services.

> *'The amount of involvement of ministers was quite extraordinary.'*
> *(Bill Burmester)*

> *'The quality of the people in the secretariat was extraordinary. It was just so hard to keep them once they got known around the place. They all seemed to be extremely intelligent and effective people, so you would lose them.' (Derek Volker)*

The government did not rely on the usual processes within the bureaucracy but used a hybrid approach, partly political and partly bureaucratic (Holub 1985: 1). A small group within DSS was set up to serve the Cabinet Subcommittee on Maintenance, called the **Maintenance Secretariat**. It was headed by Meredith Edwards. Edwards was a ministerial consultant to Brian Howe but in fact operated out of DSS as head of this secretariat and for most purposes worked as a public servant, a fairly rare arrangement at the time. Working out of DSS was important for harnessing the bureaucracy.

> **18 December 1985** This week Cabinet approved me as Ministerial Consultant to Brian Howe to work on maintenance issues heading a secretariat within DSS. Tuesday I saw Howe primarily to discuss my relationship with him, the Department and the Social Security Review. I also met that day with Don Grimes and his staff talking maintenance issues.

The Maintenance Secretariat contracted highly knowledgeable and energetic lawyers with fresh ideas, and this contributed to the success of the scheme (Edwards 1992). These people had no idea of how the bureaucracy worked and there was no time to train them in other than the basics. They were pitched against public servants who could see many problems with the scheme, yet the 'outsiders' turned these problems into challenges and came up with highly creative solutions to many complex issues. At the beginning there was little interdepartmental cooperation and some suspicion about the role of the secretariat, but with time this changed. Michael Keating, head of the Department of Finance at the time, after a meeting with Meredith Edwards instructed his officers to work more closely with the Secretariat.

> *'There was certainly resistance from the bureaucracy. There was resistance to trusting and working with the secretariat for a while because they were new faces in Canberra; their status was not completely understood . . . (Bill Burmester)*

Howe used the government bureaucracy and its processes with extraordinary insight and skill. As minister responsible for child support, having taken over the reins in February 1986, Howe asked each minister on the Cabinet Subcommittee to provide an officer to work within the secretariat. When that was resisted, it was agreed that ministers of the subcommittee should nominate 'contact' officers to work on child maintenance issues but within their host departments. These contacts met regularly with the Maintenance Secretariat, particularly before a meeting of the subcommittee.

> *'Ministers were aware that because departments were opposed to the reform, they had to persuade departments into action.'*
> *(Brian Howe)*

Papers to the Cabinet Subcommittee, prepared by the secretariat, did not go through the Cabinet Office as normal. They were seen but rarely influenced by the departmental secretary and went direct to the minister. What Howe received was a report from the secretariat after it had found out the views of departments and usually their ministers, so there were few surprises for Howe when ministers met.

> *'The IDC was a mechanism built for failure. By way of contrast, the "contacts group" gave the Maintenance Secretariat an opportunity to convince departments how they could contribute: the contacts group was problem-focused.' (Brian Howe)*

Howe was well aware of the potential of Labor backbenchers to sink his proposals. From late 1986 he therefore set up a **Subcommittee of Caucus** under the chair of Pat Giles to work on backbenchers who either thought it electorally damaging for the government to take on this issue or were NCPs themselves. The other women members of this subcommittee, Caroline Jakobson and Rosemary Crowley, became important advocates of the reforms within Caucus.

Senior DSS officials were quite strongly opposed to the child support proposal throughout, and members of the Maintenance Secretariat felt their hostility strongly. Child support reforms were seen as a 'feminist plot'; the day of a key decision by Cabinet was seen as 'a black day for Australian fathers'. In addition, DSS officials were sceptical as to whether any scheme could produce significant net revenue savings. There are many instances of DSS resistance tactics, for example using a bomb scare as an excuse to relocate the secretariat out of the DSS building:

> It was quite clear that every element of the bureaucracy was opposed to the Scheme and this is highlighted for me by an anecdote: when I was working in the Maintenance Secretariat, it was not uncommon for us at that time to receive bomb threats against the staff in the Secretariat from agitated non-custodial parents' groups. And on one occasion, we received advice through the Department of Social Security that . . . this particular threat had some merit and that we should be worried about it . . . Meredith . . . had gone off to talk to the then deputy secretary about what we should do about it . . . and he shut her up in no uncertain terms saying that he was not interested in talking about it: his concern was that we could not stay in the [Social Security] building where other departmental staff were working for more than another day. He did not care where we went or what we did but we were not to be near any of their 'real' people. (Brennan 1995: 5)

As late as December 1986, the head of the department insisted that child support activities be kept separate from other departmental activities in case the child support exercise 'fell flat on its face'. Many officials also expected public opposition to overwhelm the proposal and therefore did not take it seriously for a considerable time.

> *'There was a strong view at the higher levels that this was a load of rubbish and it would not fly. It was necessary, therefore, that it was not handled through DSS. It needed to be a separate exercise with the Minister's support . . . and a government initiative. The department was pretty bruised then by a number of recent decisions, including the assets test.' (Derek Volker)*

The **Department of Finance** cooperated with the Maintenance Secretariat in the DSS because of its interest in gaining revenue for the government. An officer was seconded to the secretariat for much of this process, which made for a close working relationship throughout the exercise. This work was invaluable in helping Cabinet come to in-principle decisions about the fundamentals of the scheme in the lead-up to the August 1986 Budget.

The position adopted by the **Department of Prime Minister and Cabinet** was not as tough as that of Finance but more revenue-

THE PLAYERS

Politicians

Bowen, Lionel	Attorney–General, 1984–90 and Deputy Prime Minister
Crowley, Rosemary	Member, Caucus Working Group on Child Support
Evans, Gareth	Attorney-General, 1983–84
Giles, Pat	Chair, Caucus Working Group on Child Support
Grimes, Don	Minister for Social Security, 1983–84; Minister for Community Services, 1984–87
Hawke, Bob	Prime Minister
Howe, Brian	Minister for Social Security
Jakobson, Caroline	Member, Caucus Working Group on Child Support
Keating, Paul	Treasurer
Ryan, Susan	Minister Assisting the Prime Minister on the Status of Women Minister for Education
Walsh, Peter	Minister for Finance

Ministerial advisers

Burns, Netta	Senior Adviser to Minister for Social Security
Edwards, Dr Meredith	Ministerial Consultant, 1986–87
Russell, Dr Don	Senior Adviser to Treasurer

Public servants

Argyll, Catherine	Head, Child Support Agency, 1996–
Boucher, Trevor	Commissioner, ATO
Brennan, Tom	Member, Maintenance Secretariat 1984 and later Ministerial Consultant to Brian Howe
Burmester, Bill	Senior officer, Department of Finance
Butler, David	Senior officer, ATO, 1993–96
Edwards, Dr Meredith	Head, Social Policy Division, DSS, May 1987–90
Finn, Mary	Senior officer, Attorney–General's Department
Gardner, Peter	Senior officer, ABS
O'Loughlin, Mary Ann	Senior official, PM&C

Roche, Michael	Branch Head, PM&C
Rose, Dennis	Principal adviser to Attorney-General, 1984–87
Scollay, Moira	Second Commissioner, Taxation Child Support Agency, ATO, 1994–97
Shiff, Deena	Member, Maintenance Secretariat
Sutton, Trevor	Senior officer, ATO, 1995–
Volker, Derek	Secretary, DSS
Williams, Neil	Senior officer on secondment from AGs to Maintenance Secretariat

Other

Disney, Julian	Head, ACOSS
Evatt, Justice Elizabeth AO	Chief Judge of the Family Court of Australia
Fogarty, Justice John	Judge of the Family Court of Australia, Chair, FLC 1983–86, Chair CSCG and CSCEAG 1986–91
Garfinkel, Prof. Irwin	Professor, Institute of Research on Poverty, University of Wisconsin
Harper, Patricia	Member of Family Law Council, Member of Single Parents and Their Child, Secretary, AIFS
Harrison, Margaret	AIFS, Observer on FLC
McDonald, Dr Peter	Deputy Director, AIFS
Troy, Pat	Head, Social Justice Project, ANU
Williams, Daryl	President, Law Council of Australia 1986–87

minded than that of DSS, and this was partly due to the personal interest of one of its staff, Mary Ann O'Loughlin. PM&C had considerable influence over process, for example whether child support issues went directly to Cabinet or through the Expenditure Review Committee (ERC). Understandably, the Maintenance Secretariat worked hard to keep PM&C officers informed of its own agenda so that PM&C decisions, as far as possible, fitted in with the secretariat's agenda.

The **Attorney-General's Department** was pulled in several directions but tended to err on the side of caution, aware of considerable lawyer opposition to any reduction in the power of the courts. It was served most ably by Mary Finn, who worked closely with Senator Bowen. Within the department was the **Office of**

Parliamentary Counsel (OPC), which contained specialists in drafting legislation.

The **Australian Taxation Office** (ATO) was, not surprisingly, quite resistant to the reforms. The prime concern of the ATO contact officer was to ensure that the scheme was administratively feasible, especially since the ATO had never been in this kind of business before. Once the ATO knew the die was cast and there was to be a Child Support Agency, its initial reaction was to get that agency as far removed as possible from itself. Later, when it was realised that there was no scope for carving off such an agency to another department, it moved to integrate the agency as far as possible into mainstream ATO functions.

Many IDCs or working parties were set up to develop the detail of policy and oversee implementation. For example, a Child Support Steering Committee was set up in 1987, consisting of DSS, AGs, ATO and the Department of Finance, with one of its main tasks to oversee the various components of legislation needed to introduce the scheme. This committee also oversaw publicity for the start of the scheme.

IDENTIFYING THE ISSUES

By the mid-1980s the need for reform was becoming urgent. Cabinet was keen to find ways of reducing the deficit, and placing more financial responsibility for children on the non-custodial parent was one possible way of saving government outlays. In addition, some ministers were concerned about worsening poverty among sole-parent families. The reform package, which in turn was part of a rethinking of the structure of the welfare system, aimed to move the system away from dependency to programs that encouraged more participation in the labour market.

PUTTING THE PROBLEM ON THE AGENDA

Parallel policy processes occurred in 1985 inside and outside government which were crucial in restarting the reform process and in shaping the reform agenda. On the outside, an influential body, the **Family Law Council** (FLC), played a pivotal role that affected the direction of reform; many of its members were long-time advocates for reform of the maintenance system, especially its chair, Justice John Fogarty. The FLC was sophisticated in its advocacy role, its use of tactics and its sense of timing in gaining government attention and favourable reaction to its proposals.

In November 1984 a paper by three FLC members, Meredith

Government and non-government activities 1985/86

June	FLC Subcommittee established on child support options	Government commissioned IDC on maintenance options
July	Fogarty (FLC) letter to AG on deficiencies of NZ scheme and FLC proposal principles	Government seeks more advice on options
November	Minister Howe obtains draft FLC report	Howe writes to PM proposing ministerial subcommittee
December	FLC reports to AG recommending formula-based administrative approach	Press statement on maintenance
February	Professor Garfinkel visit arranged by SJS; ANU and SJS workshop on child support arranged	Garfinkel lunches with ministers
First meeting of Ministerial Subcommittee

Edwards, Patricia Harper and Margaret Harrison (all of whom also had other relevant connections), was presented at a Family Law conference. The paper canvassed problems and possible solutions to child support, including the use of a formula for assessing maintenance according to the income of the NCP and its collection through the ATO by a tax or child-support levy. This idea had its origins in a proposal canvassed by Professor Garfinkel from the USA (1979) and is thought to be the first occasion on which these proposals were publicly put forward in Australia. Despite the incredulity with which the radical tax proposal was received by the law profession at the time, discussion of these ideas continued within the FLC in 1985. They gained increasing acceptance by Justice Fogarty and FLC members.

The FLC was aware that the Commonwealth Government was considering many options for reform and that it was disposed towards a scheme similar to the New Zealand Liable Parent Contribution Scheme (NZ LPCS). The FLC saw this as too narrow a solution and one fraught with dangers, particularly the possibility that the maintenance collected would go directly into government revenue despite the evidence which showed how poor sole parents were.

The chair of the FLC, aware of what was going on in government,

wrote to the Attorney-General in July 1985 pointing out the deficiencies of the NZ LPCS and advising him of the goals and principles
that his council believed should underlie any scheme. The main goals
espoused were to provide adequate support for children of separated
parents and to ensure that parents share equitably in the support of
their children. At this time the FLC acted strategically by setting up
a subcommittee to investigate proposals contained in the paper by
Edwards and associates (1985). In December 1985 the FLC submitted its reform proposals to the Attorney-General (FLC 1985). The
Council proposed that child maintenance should be set up by means
of a simple formula, applied in the first instance administratively
rather than judicially, and collected from the non-custodial parent
by automatic witholding of income through the taxation system.

Meanwhile, inside the government bureaucracy in mid-1985 there
were several meetings of a Commonwealth IDC which examined
options for reform of the maintenance system. These included not
only the NZ LPCS but also modifications to the recommendations in
the Attorney-General's Department report. The real driving force at
this stage was the government's desire for increased revenue, but
ministers could not agree on which of the many options to progress.

Social Security Minister Brian Howe was particularly impressed
with the clear articulation of the problem by the FLC; it convinced
him that he needed to take a leadership role on policy direction.
When he read the FLC's draft report around September 1985, he
realised how closely he identified with its principles and objectives,
especially improving the position of children in poverty. Soon afterwards he put it to Prime Minister Hawke that ministers should be
more involved in the process of reform.

Howe wrote to Hawke in November 1985 proposing to set up
a Cabinet Subcommittee on Maintenance to examine the child
maintenance issue (see above). Around this time a significant decision was taken when Howe and the Treasurer, Paul Keating, decided
that reform could benefit both revenue and sole parents. They were
aware that many in the Commonwealth bureaucracy were opposed
to the scheme—no government agency wanted the task of collecting
and enforcing maintenance, let alone assessing an appropriate level
of payment. DSS was particularly strong on this point.

*'Child Support was the "hard stuff" to counter the "soft stuff"
—the family allowance supplement. This was the way to get
through to Keating and Walsh.' (Brian Howe)*

An unusual feature of this major reform was that there was no
significant lobby group advocating it. It was very much a policy
driven from within government, with the exception of the role played

by the FLC. Minister Howe, in particular, with the support of the FLC, redefined the objectives away from just saving money, and this enabled the reforms to progress.

ARTICULATING THE PROBLEM

In this case, the problem was easy to articulate: why should a child suffer financially just because its parents chose no longer to live together? It was also easy to appeal to taxpayers: why should they foot the bill just because parents decide to live separately? Unlike many other policy development processes that struggle to articulate the problem and gain its acceptance and eventually stall, the problem was expanded beyond the need for government revenue to include the needs of children. The adverse financial impact on children whose parents had separated was reiterated many times during the reform process (and refined in the light of data), as was the capacity of many NCPs to pay more than they were paying.

In February 1986 the Social Justice Project (SJP) headed by Patrick Troy, in which Meredith Edwards was working on child support reform, hosted the visit to Australia of Professor Irwin Garfinkel, from the Institute of Poverty Research at the University of Wisconsin. Garfinkel was the architect of a pilot child-support program being tested in the State of Wisconsin and which the FLC, in 1985, adapted to form its own proposal. The formula eventually adopted by the government closely followed the Wisconsin model.

> *23 February 1986* To lunch on Wednesday at the Lobby with five of the six ministers of the Cabinet Subcommittee: Howe, Grimes, Bowen, Walsh and Ryan. At a crucial early stage, Howe asked Garfinkel to explain to Bowen his proposal. Garfinkel held the attention of the five ministers for over ten minutes with his three-part proposal: the standard (formula), automatic income withholding, and child benefits. Intelligent questions were asked, particularly by Bowen. On to meet Kate Legge of the *Age* for an interview. She clearly got the impression from Garfinkel that the ministers were interested. On to see Grimes and Howe popped in. His main concern was the 16-year-old boy from a low-income family and not wanting to saddle him for life for his misdemeanours. 4.30 p.m. appointment with Bowen, who was 'knocked over' by Garfinkel's ideas.
>
> Rung on Friday by AG's to say Bowen really was taken by Garfinkel and had asked his head of department to meet

> Garfinkel and make maintenance a high priority. So if G. did nothing else, he has won over Bowen and so there are four on side. Not bad!

Garfinkel's visit brought a degree of publicity to child maintenance issues and raised understanding within the bureaucracy and the community on some of the more complex issues. The fact that senior ministers made themselves available to meet Garfinkel is an indication of the serious commitment being then given to child support by the government (Holub 1989: 15). Garfinkel impressed ministers with his clear presentation of what could be achieved. This is an obvious illustration of the overlap between the earlier and later stages in the policy cycle, since Garfinkel was promoting a solution as much as gaining acceptance of the problem.

POLICY ANALYSIS

Few policy development processes could have thrown up as many difficult and sensitive issues for analysis as did the child support reforms. There was a vast array of complex political, legal, administrative and other problems, crossing many portfolio interests. For the desired objectives to be achieved, it was necessary (but by no means sufficient) to undertake as comprehensive and rigorous a policy analysis as possible. What follows focuses on policy analysis in 1986 and 1987, although another and overlapping period of analysis occurred in 1987 and 1988 once Cabinet had come to in-principle decisions and needed them spelt out.

The policy analysis stage is where bureaucrats can play a crucial role. In this case senior ministers were the pivot. Ministers had their own separate agendas and their expectations were bound to conflict. Howe nevertheless obtained an unusual degree of cooperation between finance and welfare ministers, and, at least initially, the Attorney-General, because the scheme took pressure off the Family Court.

Once the dual objectives of achieving revenue and assisting sole parents had been defined, the main source of tension among ministers was keeping the balance between them. Howe and Ryan were most concerned to improve the position of sole-parent families. Keating and Walsh mainly wanted savings, and so supported harsher options, but both also had an eye on equitable treatment of parents. Bowen wanted savings but also a system that reduced the burden on the Family Court, while Grimes appeared to want changes but more focus on an effective collection and enforcement system than on assessment.

In July 1986 Cabinet considered the final report of the Cabinet Subcommittee and came to in-principle decisions. This allowed a discussion paper to be released in October to start the formal consultation process. As is evident in other public policy case studies, once in-principle decisions were made by ministers on the framework and key principles of the reform, much more detailed policy analysis was required before legislation could be drafted and the policies implemented.

DATA AND RESEARCH

From its beginning in February 1986, the Maintenance Secretariat adopted a systematic approach to collecting information. This was necessary to counter opposition. The scheme was open to attack on many fronts, especially the fairly widespread belief (in DSS at least) that insufficient revenue would be raised because most NCPs were believed to have low incomes. There was also the belief (among feminists, for example) that a significant proportion of unmarried mothers would not want to declare the father of their child. The Maintenance Secretariat was constantly using data, including from overseas, to counter such arguments.

A rigorous process was then used to determine the revenue and distributional impact of the scheme, especially identifying winners and losers. For example, early in the process a meeting was held between the secretariat and the Department of Finance to agree on costings/revenue and income distribution assumptions so as to prevent arguments later. Early agreement with Finance on financial parameters was not a common bureaucratic practice at the time but had been followed successfully in developing AUSTUDY (see Chapter 2). The arrangement was that once assumptions were agreed, they would not be changed unless significant new data emerged to make change necessary.

> *19 April 1986* Saw ABS Tuesday and realised how bad our database was. A real worry. Peter Gardner of ABS was so enthusiastic and helpful and could see I needed new data by Friday. It came minus a crucial piece on income ranges. So today (Saturday) an ABS guy will give us the remaining data.

An important piece of unavailable data that was needed early in the exercise was the income of NCPs, so that the likely net revenue to be generated by the scheme could be estimated. The Maintenance Secretariat approached the ABS in April 1986 for urgent assistance with this missing data, and the result made the revenue figures look robust. It is difficult to know how much ministers' interest in the exercise would have waned had the error in that data, discovered by the ABS five months later, been known earlier, since the corrected data reduced revenue estimates by over 30 per cent.

A good illustration of the depth of research was the data-gathering and analysis around determining the costs of raising children, and therefore the percentage used in the formula to determine what proportion of NCPs' income was to be paid. Overseas information, particularly from the USA, was mined, and debates occurred with key researchers over the appropriate method to reflect the costs of a child in the formula. Commonly, the figure of 20 per cent of income was the cost of the first child for a large range of income. In the end, the percentages chosen were arbitrary and erred on the low side of the costs of children, bowing to political factors.

Little data was available at the time of the AG's inquiry in 1983 into maintenance enforcement. Relevant and timely data was needed later to ensure that policy-makers and the broader public understood the dimensions of the problem of sole-parent poverty and the role in this of the lack of child maintenance payments. An important body providing useful data was the **Australian Institute of Family Studies** (AIFS). In 1985, for example, it published the influential *Economic Consequences of Marital Breakdown*, written by its deputy director, Dr Peter McDonald, which demonstrated convincingly the low 'coverage' of custodians who had maintenance orders or agreements, the persistently low levels of maintenance orders where they existed, and the low payment rate.

RESOLVING KEY QUESTIONS

19 April 1986 We had a victory this week: a letter from the PM accepting our timetable and the need to consult. He also now has the message that there is no money in maintenance in the 1986/87 financial year. Looks like Michael Roche and Mary Ann O'Loughlin have been briefing appropriately.

A successful stage in the process leading to the new Child Support Scheme was to ensure that ministers first confronted key questions or issues that were potentially contentious, rather than starting by debating difficult options such as where to locate the collection agency (this was deliberately left till last). At the outset Howe had determined that the first meeting of the Cabinet Subcommittee would identify areas of agreement, leaving more contentious matters to later meetings. Ministers then progressively confronted harder decisions; if they had dealt up front with harder issues, such as where to locate the agency, the debate would have quickly reached impasse.

In retrospect, one of the difficulties faced by the 1985 child maintenance IDCs referred to earlier was developing too many options, without ministers first discussing what basic elements they wanted in a reform package. Each option tended to reflect the interests of a single department, with a main issue of contention being which department would house the collection and enforcement agency.

The first set of key issues confronted by ministers from February 1986 were whether to

- use an administrative or court-based system
- use a formula
- use the ATO for collection and enforcement with automatic deduction from PAYE, or
- go beyond pensioners and include non-pensioners in the scheme.

In relation to the first issue, at a Family Law conference in June 1986, Justice Fogarty said he had for many years believed the solution to ineffective enforcement of maintenance was through the courts. But he went on to say:

> I am now persuaded, contrary to my initial reaction to this matter, that:
> (a) the present system is incapable of dealing with the problem and no amount of adaptation of it will meet the problem;
> (b) a largely administrative rather than a legal response to this problem is now called for. (Fogarty 1986)

Over the course of policy development, the enthusiasm of ministers waxed and waned. This was the case particularly with Bowen, who earlier had been an enthusiastic supporter of a simpler system. Around the middle of the year he realised that even though government might benefit from more revenue, most sole parents would remain on a pension. Grimes and Walsh also lost interest over time; increasingly Walsh could see that he would not get the savings he wanted in the August 1987 Budget, and Grimes worried about the impact on non-custodial parents.

The extent of ministers' involvement in deliberations was unusual. Perhaps previously failed attempts to get maintenance reform led to greater determination to find a solution, with the six members of the Cabinet Subcommittee meeting many times, particularly in the first half of 1986. They oversaw a fast pace of policy development, from their first meeting in early February 1986, when their modus operandi was agreed, to the adoption of principles for the scheme as well as its fundamentals just three months later in May. By June further decisions had been made on the divisive issue of which agency should collect and enforce maintenance.

> *4 May 1986* Friday was the day ministers met for their second substantial meeting. Saw the Minister at 8.45 a.m. to go over our strategy. Into the Cabinet room at 9 a.m., but no one there. Susan Ryan soon arrived and hoped the meeting would not be too long; Bowen was on his way from Government House. Don Russell appeared acting as Treasurer, who was ill; Don Grimes, we were told, had Senate duty and did not intend to come out. Walsh was not to be located but turned up soon after calling for aspirin . . . Meeting finished around 10 a.m. In that time we had 100 per cent success on decisions the Minister called for . . .
>
> Last week the secretariat worked on the Interim Report ministers have to give to Cabinet. Very tight timetable. We finished it Friday arvo and Monday it goes to the department, Howe, and then to ministers to be considered by them next Wednesday.

Throughout the process of obtaining in-principle decisions in 1986, the Maintenance Secretariat produced regular progress reports for ministers indicating what had been decided and what issues remained on the table. Decisions on these basic issues were endorsed in principle by Cabinet in mid-July 1986 (see below), which meant that the main planks of the scheme could be announced in the August 1986 Budget. Cabinet at that time also noted a list of dispositions on policy and some second-order issues which remained to be resolved.

> *11 May 1986* Wednesday was the meeting of ministers to endorse the interim report to Cabinet, which is due to go tomorrow. Meeting due to start at 9.30 a.m. . . . Into Cabinet Room at 10 a.m. But Grimes had gone by then and Bowen preoccupied by [a crisis]. Chased around to get Bowen, Keating and Ryan. All agreed within the hour.
>
> Friday had a 'contacts' meeting. Depressing. Tax Office predictable and not saying definitely when their paper would be due despite a meeting of ministers calling for it last week. Don Russell from Treasurer's office said he would get it by 9 May. After the meeting, Deena Shiff and I thought through tactics and decided to see the Minister a.m. Monday and to seek information from ATO in a neutral way, putting the issue of the location of the agency, at this stage, to one side.

The last and hardest decision (made in May) was the location of the collection agency, which was a compromise decision amounting to good politics more than to good policy. Howe initially wanted the most efficient process by having the collection, enforcement and distribution of child support to take place under the one roof of the ATO. However, conscious of the extreme opposition of the ATO to any involvement in the first place, Paul Keating as Treasurer, and Minister responsible for the ATO, sought and received agreement from Brian Howe to involve the DSS in the distribution of payments to sole parents. Being prepared to compromise but when and on what is a key skill of politicians, which Howe exercised on this occasion to good effect, despite briefing to him to do otherwise.

> 'I recall Keating calling me to his office to say, "You are someone with a social conscience—can't you do something to help us here?" I replied that the Tax Office could manage the collection function but was not up to distributing payments.' (Trevor Boucher)

The order in which key issues were debated by ministers was important in getting final agreement to the framework of the scheme. For example, as noted before, had the issue about location of the agency been faced earlier, or the contentious issue of income testing and the related question of distribution of savings from the scheme been confronted before the Budget, then the division among ministers would most likely have interfered with their achieving radical reform.

The government announced its in-principle position in August, just six months from the first meeting of the Cabinet Subcommittee:

> The Government intends to replace [the] system of judicial discretion with a legislative formula administered by a child support agency under the control of the Commissioner of Taxation. Mr Howe said the precise details of the formula had not yet been decided. ('Major Reform . . .', Press Release, 19 August 1986)

Lead-up to Cabinet in-principle decisions, May–June 1986

11 May 1986 We really are into a difficult round on location and income-testing issues. Excellent decisions so far but not on the contentious ones. The more I can draw in the department [DSS] the less it all rests on my shoulders.

1 June 1986 It is an incredible and frightening responsibility to have a major say over such a complex policy issue with only a slim chance of it all working out and real dangers that sole parents may gain little. But I like the challenge of handling it and the step-by-step attempting to find a way through. I am impatient with the detail but realise the need for it . . .

9 June 1986 Meeting of ministers Thursday night left me exhausted. Meant to start at 7 p.m. Walsh had to go into Senate at 8 p.m. Keating not available. Started nearer 7.30 p.m. Walsh went out but back in half an hour or so. Grimes out for a while and back. Bowen there throughout. Most undisciplined discussion going all over the place . . . The role of Cabinet note-takers is interesting. They need watching like a hawk.

15 June 1986 Thursday called 'contacts' meeting to go over an ATO proposal. Very interesting trying to work out what game ATO is playing. Looks to me like they are establishing a case for a separate agency even if under their umbrella so that if that argument is accepted, they can quickly hive it off onto some other body.

29 June 1986 Ministers met Tuesday night in the Cabinet room. Officials in for first time. Deena hilarious and like a puppy dog passing notes [to me]—not to pass on to Minister necessarily but expressing her overflowing feelings, like 'this is going from bad to worse' . . . Hilarious to watch Keating huddled around two ATO officials plus his personal adviser. Apparently he said afterwards, 'They want us to do the shitwork and collect the money and then they want to spend it on welfare'. A bad meeting but not disastrous.

DEVELOPING OPTIONS

Several options arose after ministers made their in-principle decisions, for example whether the scheme should be retrospective or how to test custodial parents' income and the appropriate formula to use. The first was resolved before the discussion paper was issued in October. Income-testing options took longer (well into 1987 and interrupted by the election in that year). In some ways the latter was the hardest major decision because it was to affect the income of sole parents as well as government revenue. As would be expected, ministers were divided on this throughout.

Before these and other options could be rigorously analysed, however, agreement was needed on a set of criteria on which to base the analysis of options. For example, in assessing different types of formulae options were assessed according to the following criteria:

- whether there was fair treatment of NCPs, especially those on low incomes

- the work-disincentive impact on NCPs
- simplicity in administration
- financial implications.

In early 1987 Cabinet decided not to make final decisions on the formula issue but instead referred the formula to a **Child Support Consultative Group** (CSCG) as part of the development of Stage 2 of the scheme (see below). Several options were considered by this group in a consultative framework (see CSCG 1988).

When the Maintenance Secretariat advised Howe early in 1987 on the timing of reforms, particularly whether or not to bring in the reforms in two stages, they used several explicit criteria to assess the timing options:

- the politics of introducing legislation before the election due that year
- the likely community response
- the impact of staging on eventual implementation
- the effect on other government activities, for example the planned 'families package'.

CONSULTATION

In any consultation process it is important to ascertain the power of lobby groups and to understand their internal politics. Lobby groups, in turn, need to understand political and bureaucratic processes if they want to make a difference. In this case the FLC was more aware of what to do to get the proposals onto the agenda than was the relatively influential Law Council of Australia. The latter did have an influence in deferring but not stopping the introduction of a formula.

Consultation can and should be continuous throughout the development of policy and into the implementation stage. This was certainly the case here. There was continuous consultation both within and outside government, including consultations on quite specific issues. There was also constant contact between Minister Howe and the Caucus backbench committee headed by Pat Giles. This group was always well briefed, by the secretariat and others, especially on sensitive issues around the formula.

The main consultation on the scheme as a whole occurred in October 1986 on the basis of a discussion paper tabled by the Cabinet Subcommittee and released soon after the principles of the scheme had been announced: 'While the broad outline of the scheme was announced in the [1986/87] Budget, many detailed decisions will not be taken until public submissions have been received on the discussion paper' (Howe, 8 October 1986: 2).

> **22 June 1986** From now on, [it is a] matter of making sure maintenance exercise stays on the rails. Clear-cut tasks ahead: writing discussion paper and consulting. Then really over to legislative drafters and administrators.

Having made in-principle decisions by the middle of 1986, ministers did not want these decisions undone. They therefore endorsed a discussion paper which assumed the major planks of the scheme as effectively 'non-negotiable' and sought views on 'second-order, but complex' issues. For example, in a formula,

- how should the income of the custodial parent be treated?
- how should custodial parents be treated if they refused to provide information about the non-custodial parent?
- how was paternity to be established when that was in dispute?

The Maintenance Secretariat advised Howe against public consultations as undertaken by the Maintenance Inquiry in 1984, preferring smaller bilateral discussions which would attract less publicity and were less likely to go off the rails. Bilateral consultations went ahead, and were conducted within the framework of the discussion paper. Several lobby groups criticised the tight timing of the consultation process, which was given barely two weeks between release of the discussion paper and the start of formal consultations and with only one month for the consultations themselves.

Despite the limited time to prepare, over 300 written submissions were received and a broad range of groups was consulted. There was strong general support for the principles of the scheme, including agreement that the current system of determining levels of child maintenance had little relationship to either capacity to pay or the needs of the child. There was broad agreement to place greater priority on the responsibility of parents to support their children whether or not they happened to be living with them.

The reaction of editorial writers was heartening to the government (e.g. *Age* 13 October 1986, *Adelaide Advertiser* 10 October 1986). Groups representing both women and welfare interests were generally supportive of the government's proposed initiatives at this time. In most cases, however, support was conditional on improvements to the financial position of sole parents and the lack of an adverse financial effect on children where the custodial parent chose not to provide information about the NCP (Edwards 1986a). Fear of the scheme being a government savings option was another concern. There was also opposition to the need for sole parents to take maintenance action to become eligible for the sole-parent pension.

There was understandable opposition from NCPs, who wanted their payments conditional on obtaining access to their children. The national president of the Lone Fathers Association, for example, released 'An Address to the Nation' on the issue (Holub 1989: 21–2). Differences emerged also on the relative responsibility of NCPs to first and later children. It was constantly emphasised that any formula should not reduce second families to poverty. This became a crucial variable in future analysis.

As would be expected, lawyers were particularly concerned to ensure that a formula was capable of responding to the circumstances of each individual case. The Law Council of Australia considered that a formula for assessment would not take proper account of the financial situation of parents and that this was more properly the province of the courts.

It is interesting to note that while there was quite strong opposition from several lobby groups to the proposed radical changes, few detailed alternatives were put forward by them. In other words, it could be argued that interest groups had potential for a lot more influence than they showed. In part this could have been because it was fairly late in the piece that many major players, inside and outside government, believed that the vision of reform held by Minister Howe might be realised.

Within a week of consultations finishing, the Maintenance Secretariat had completed a summary document on the results for the Cabinet Subcommittee. The secretariat then produced a publicly available report on consultations (Edwards 1986a).

The Cabinet Subcommittee revised their position on several matters after they heard the outcome of formal consultations. They recommended to Cabinet, for example, softening the treatment of custodial parents who refused to provide information about NCPs, different treatment of custodial parents' incomes than proposed in the discussion paper, and measures to protect the financial position of NCPs, especially where there was a second family to support. The consultations also drew attention to the need for an extensive education campaign to accompany the introduction of the scheme, a matter which the Cabinet Subcommittee took on board.

At this time there was much publicity in the press about the reforms, with the response of editorial writers being generally positive. Key journalists, such as Kate Legge in the *Age*, having been kept as informed as possible throughout the process of reform, were important communicators with the public about facts, research findings and government objectives.

Another major consultation on formula issues took place through the Child Support Consultative Group, whose report was delivered to government in 1988. The CSCG was set up by the government in May 1987 and chaired by Justice Fogarty. It set out the administrative process for the scheme and details of the formula for assessing what NCPs should pay. Its membership was from various interest groups that covered custodial and non-custodial parent groups, welfare groups, employers, the ATO, and lawyers. It published a unanimous report on the formula in May 1988. Reaction to this report was again generally positive, but the Law Council was particularly opposed.

Because the Law Council's position was so strident, and because it was unable to compromise, its effectiveness with government on formula issues was reduced; both Government and Opposition effectively ignored its views. The council failed in two ways. First, it underestimated its constituents, for example family lawyers in the suburbs, who may have had some concerns but were not as opposed as their executive body was making out. Second, it acted arrogantly, for example opposing a formula outright when the government had already decided there would be a formula and had asked the CSCG to examine what type was most appropriate. In refusing to put a submission to the CSCG, the Law Council ultimately lost much credibility.

'[The Law Council] used the political route, attempting to influence politicians without wanting to be part of the process the politicians had set up. They therefore sidelined themselves.'
(John Fogarty)

MOVING TOWARDS DECISIONS

The formal consultation process held late in 1986 alerted lobby groups to the seriousness of the government's intention to pursue reform, especially the use of formula assessment. Early in 1987 the scheme appeared to be in jeopardy: press headlines reflected the fact that the government was backing off from the reforms, particularly in the light of public criticisms from the Law Council of Australia. Its president, Daryl Williams QC, asserted that 'the assessment of maintenance . . . should continue to be the responsibility of the courts' (*Age* 24 January 1987).

In January 1987 an article by David Clarke in the *Australian Financial Review* raised concerns about the 'unintended consequences' of the scheme. Drawing heavily on concerns expressed by Lone

Fathers Association and the Law Council, Clarke drew attention to how vulnerable the scheme appeared:

> There has been far too little critical public discussion of the document Child Support, issued by the Cabinet Sub-Committee on Maintenance, which proposes that maintenance payments be collected through a Maintenance Agency, according to a rigid formula. Instead, the only Australian who will remain unaffected by decisions about to be made by Cabinet on this matter will be tax exempt celebrants.
>
> Some Canberra femocrats will undoubtedly reach for their marking pliers after reading the following. However, the questions raised below deserve clear, unequivocal answers from Mr Howe, the Minister for Social Security, and those responsible for the discussion document. (*AFR*, 13 January 1987)

What followed in Clarke's article was a series of questions that no doubt would have been uppermost in the minds of some NCPs: will the income of the custodial parent be considered in setting maintenance payments? what about the self-employed? will unwed mothers be obliged to name the father of their children?

Senator Grimes, acting for Minister Howe while he was on leave, and prompted by Clarke's article, expressed his concerns about the proposed reforms to the Prime Minister. Grimes was concerned at the timing of the legislation; he did not want it to be passed before the election due that year, especially because of the impact it might have on NCPs' income and the second family, which by this stage was a matter of public concern. He also identified unforeseen consequences of bringing in a formula which needed far more work. A particular concern was the impact of the formula on middle-income NCPs.

> *17 January 1987* Clarke's article looked more penetrating than it was, but it obviously has made many people nervous of 'unintended consequences'.
>
> Netta Burns from Grimes's office told me on Tuesday that Grimes was going to see the PM about several issues and to express his concern about where child support was going. I realised there was little I could do . . . Grimes did articulate his concerns to me: primarily that we were heading towards slugging the NCP too much, particularly if the NCP had a second family, and more so if the custodial parent was well off. He expressed his concerns about timing and his preference not to do anything until after the next election. By the end of the day it was clear we needed to work up a paper on timing and do some work on custodial parents' income and financial resources. I cannot keep up this pace, but survival of the scheme is at stake right now.

Minister rang in from holidays. He was optimistic and not too concerned about nervousness of his colleagues or press reports (some of which he had seen). He pointed out the importance of the child support exercise for the acceptability of the families measures.

24 January 1987 At 4.30 p.m. on Wednesday I saw the Minister . . . At the meeting was Derek Volker and Netta Burns. I took Neil Williams and Tom Brennan. It was an excellent meeting because the Minister had not only thought through the timing options but developed them while we were there.

Brian Howe returned from leave in January 1987 to heated political and media debate on the future of child support reforms. He attempted to save the scheme, which was by then in danger of foundering, by setting to work on options to set up the scheme in two stages.

7 February 1987 Monday was the meeting of ministers . . . I have not gone to a meeting of ministers before so unsure of the likely result . . . Howe wanted to get in and out of the meeting as quickly as possible and achieve the recommendations that were already before ministers. Howe let all ministers have a say then succinctly summarised the decisions he wanted. Took about one and a half hours. Excellent result, given that we had already been prepared to compromise.

14 February 1987 Heard that Bowen saw Elizabeth Evatt and at that meeting he told her that he and Walsh were going to stop the child support project—to alter marginally the Family Law Act and to hold off the collection agency until after the election! Tom told me and tears came to my eyes. For the first time I realised how you can slave your guts out for absolutely no result.

Howe realised that this was a time when the scheme was most vulnerable to opposition and could be lost, or at least confined only to reform of collection and enforcement procedures. He showed great skill in judging what and when to compromise. Had he decided early in 1987 to pursue the reforms all at once, as originally planned, there is little doubt that there would have emerged only incremental changes to existing arrangements. At the same time, Stage 2 eventuated partly because the Minister (and those working with him), while attending to detail and compromising as needed, never lost sight of the vision that was driving the reform, despite the difficulty of the decisions. In an ever-threatening environment, Howe saved the totality of his desired reforms.

> Minister for Social Security, Brian Howe, today announced a new system of support to give the children of separated parents a better start in life.
>
> 'These children are among the poorest groups in our society—70% of parents, no longer living with their children, do not pay regular support,' Mr Howe said.
>
> 'The new child support system will
>
> 1. Set up a Child Support Agency, under the control of the Commissioner of Taxation, to assess child support obligations according to a legislative formula.
> 2. Enable parents to take appeals against Agency decisions to court and to ask the court to exercise discretion in contentious cases.
> 3. Collect maintenance through the Agency's tax collection mechanisms:
>   — pay as you earn taxpayers will have support deducted from their wages;
>   — self employed people will make monthly payments to the Agency;
> 4. Distribute child support through the Department of Social Security.' (News Release, 23 March 1987)

There were many other changes to the original conception of the scheme at various points in policy development. For example, after the consultation process it became clear to several government agencies that it would be difficult to establish the proposed reforms by relying on Commonwealth tax powers, so moves were made to rely more on referral of powers from the states over ex-nuptial children. But the government did not resile from its decision to use a formula to determine child support payments. It announced the details of its radical scheme in March 1987 and also that, while there would be a formula, the CSCG would recommend what that formula should be. The March statement bowed to lobby group opposition and the results of its consultations by announcing publicly that the scheme would proceed in two stages:

> Consultations here in Australia also showed widespread support for the reform—but the Government has recognised the need to sensitively shape this new system which will affect so many families at a very emotional time in their lives. (Howe 1987a)

> For this reason the Australian Government has decided on a two stage reform to allow a smooth transition to the new scheme. (Howe 1987b)

29 March 1987 An exciting and eventful week . . . Monday of this week was when Cabinet was scheduled to discuss child support as well as family assistance . . . At 4 p.m. met the Minister with additional briefing and spent around three-quarters of an hour going through briefing prior to Cabinet meeting . . . Told Minister of Bowen's position. Tom and I waited until Minister came out of Cabinet around 6.45 p.m., when he said all decisions had been passed! He had not raised discussion on a parliamentary statement (containing details of Stage 2) because it could cause controversy. I said, but . . . Stage 2 . . . was it supported? He repeated he had got all decisions except the start date of the scheme. I said I would ring PM&C to check the decision. Minister thought that a good idea. It was hard to take in the fact that we had what we wanted! We had won! Rang Michael Roche at PM&C and all OK. Back to the office to make changes to the Statement to reflect no starting date announcement . . .

On Wednesday happened to run into a key senior officer. What did he think of the announcement? 'Don't know; haven't read the papers' and then he proceeded to say it was a black day for separated Australian males and it was all going too far the women's way! . . . No congratulations from the department.

It is a marvellous victory, but we are only too aware that it is by no means over yet. But we did do the almost impossible because the attitude in the bureaucracy was 'it wouldn't get up', 'it is too complex' etc. etc., showing how much a determined minister can do with the right doses and quality of bureaucratic support.

IMPLEMENTATION

26 July 1987 Tuesday with Derek Volker and others while they told Tom and me that they could not see how child support would work from the DSS end.

It is clear that 'the boys' are out to get me and the sharpened knives were very clear this week, particularly the last few days. The boys are using the weekend child support exercise to nail my coffin—we made a couple of errors [over the weekend] in our calculations.

In any good policy-making process, implementation issues are taken into account as policy is developed. One hard judgment any analyst needs to make is the ease with which potential policies can be implemented, particularly if those responsible for implementation err on the side of caution, as they usually do. There is no doubt that had those implementing policy in DSS and ATO, for example, been listened to rather than challenged, the scheme would not have emerged. Conversely, it could be argued that many of the implementation issues of today would have been easier to deal with had they been more clearly anticipated when the scheme was being developed.

Policy analysts also need to remember that the implementation stage can often lead to a move away from original objectives and intentions. Child support was no exception.

Towards the end of 1986, and well into 1987, several implementation committees were established to address issues such as property and maintenance, constitutional issues around whether child support could be a tax, administrative options, and costings of setting up and running the agency. Different departments chaired different committees and each committee reported to the contacts group.

MAJOR ISSUES

Two key issues arose early in the implementation process. The first related to resources. The ATO played the 'resources game' hard and made what some regarded as excessive bids for dollars for implementation. Much time was spent in negotiation between Finance, the ATO and the Maintenance Secretariat on what was a protracted resource issue.

The second key issue was timing. In the face of a complex policy process, the Maintenance Secretariat faced the constant difficulty of getting departments to deliver to an agreed but tight timeframe. The secretariat ensured that ministers agreed which department should deliver what and by when, while Cabinet provided authority to the secretariat to put pressure on departments. Further, in its regular reports to the Cabinet Subcommittee, the secretariat indicated when pieces of work were behind schedule. Sometimes these issues were taken to the Minister so he could talk to his colleagues. Getting priority for child support legislation through the OPC before the 1987 election was of real concern.

Decision-makers normally want the program to start as soon as possible, especially when there are savings to be tapped. Implementers try to stall, if for no other reason than to ensure that implementation is done well. In this case the start of the scheme was delayed several times. The ATO kept pointing to unintended consequences of a starting date for the scheme that was too soon.

21 February 1987 ATO seems to be playing big games—Tom said to me that at first they tried to ditch the agency, so deliberately kept it at arm's length from ATO. When they realised that was not going to happen, they decided to merge child support activities as much as possible into ATO and then debt recovery etc. priority would be on large tax debts and not child support arrears.

Tom was here this morning saying that DSS is not taking it seriously and sees ATO as out to get as much of the resources as possible for their own operations. Tom will get support via newspapers, and Julian Disney [then president of ACOSS] is writing to members of the subcommittee and to Hawke.

Detailed development of policy was impossible without cross-agency collaboration and cooperation. Once it was clear from the budget announcement of August 1986 that there was to be a Child Support Scheme planned to start in 1997/98, much detailed policy and legislative work was required involving, in particular, the ATO and the Departments of Social Security, Attorney-General's and Finance.

THE LEGISLATIVE PHASE

The development of the Child Support Scheme relied heavily on the policy instrument of legislation. This therefore meant relying heavily on the drafters of the legislation in the Office of Parliamentary Counsel in the Attorney-General's Department.

Back in July 1986 the Maintenance Secretariat was given the role of coordinating and developing legislation. The original aim of ministers was to have legislation finalised by February 1987. The secretariat chaired regular meetings of a Legislation and Policy Coordination Group while the consultations were occurring in October 1986. Departments reported to this group after having mapped out their division of responsibilities systematically by task, by type of legislation, and with timelines.

The group deliberated intensively on a 'narrative' of the whole scheme, which illustrated the proposed operation of the scheme as a basis for drafting instructions to the OPC. Early in 1987 it became clear that the complexity of the legislation was likely to delay the legislative timetable.

'Originally we tried to base Commonwealth powers on its constitutional tax power. But there was reluctance by ministers to do that . . . so in the end powers were referred to the Commonwealth Parliament from the States over ex-nuptial children.' (Dennis Rose)

What is often missed in discussions of the policy development framework is the role of the OPC, and the people who draft legislation. They can be placed under enormous time pressures by politicians, but in the process they can exert influence on the policy outcome.

In December 1987 federal parliament passed the first of three pieces of legislation that were necessary to implement Stage 1 of the scheme, namely amendments to the *Family Law Act 1975*, *Family Law (Amendment) Act 1977*, which came into operation in April 1988. The second piece of legislation was the *Child Support Act 1988*. The third, *Social Security and Veterans' Entitlement (Maintenance Income Test) Amendment Act 1988*, also operated from June 1988.

PUBLICITY

Support from the general public was strengthened by a well-planned publicity campaign from 1986. Financial protection of children received public support, but there were some more difficult issues emerging in the press, for example whether the scheme would be retrospective and how much NCPs would need to pay; unfortunately, until the formula was decided, the latter question was not answerable.

Early in 1987 ministers agreed to a coordinated campaign across departments. DSS did not want to take the coordination responsibility, so the Maintenance Secretariat coordinated the work of a **Child Support Publicity Group** which had representatives on it not only from DSS but also the Family Court, Attorney-General's, the ATO and the Department of Sport, Recreation and Tourism (it had responsibility at the time for all government advertising). This group briefed public relations agencies on a communications strategy for the scheme and put recommendations to the Cabinet Subcommittee in the run-up to the start of Stage 1 (DSS 1994: 21f.).

> The consideration of Public Relations issues from the start as an integral part of the Scheme's introduction, and the appointment of a Public Relations consultancy relatively early in the process, were valuable factors in contributing to the successes that have been achieved. (Lee Patterson & Associates 1988: 12)

> *'We tend to forget about the importance of publicity: it looked as if the whole thing could founder. The public relations process was extraordinarily successful. One of the important things about it was the emphasis put on actually helping the children, which really got the community on side.' (Derek Volker)*

The publicity campaign had explicit objectives. These were not just to inform and obtain public support for the new system, but to

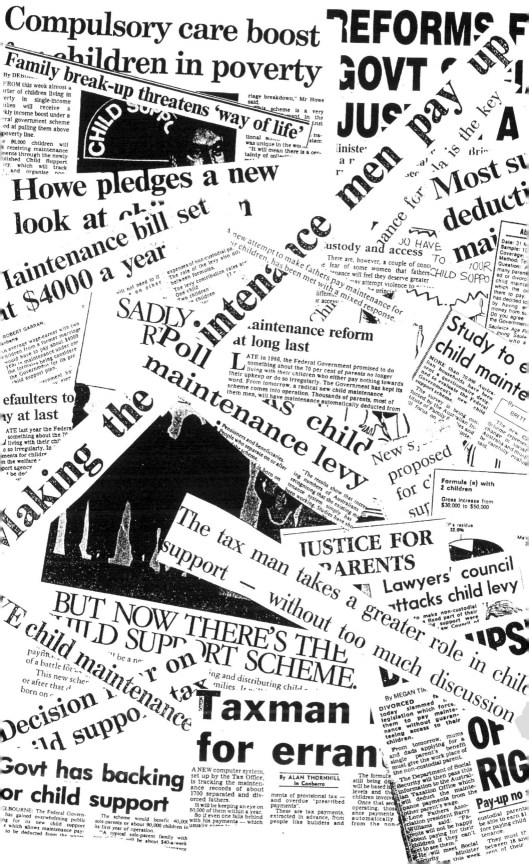

The press

This reform initiative was the focus of much publicity through-out its development (see, for example, the article by David Clarke in the *AFR* in January 1987 mentioned on p. 80 above). However there was particular press interest on 25 March 1987 immediately after Minister Howe announced the intention of the government to introduce the scheme in two stages. Several journalists who had been following the scheme reported on the proposals, the exact nature of which was still to be determined (e.g. Robert Garran of the *Age*, 'Agency to levy child support' (p. 1) and 'Maintenance bill set at $4000 a year' (p. 6); Louise O'Callaghan of the *Sydney Morning Herald*, 'Crackdown on maintenance dodgers'; and Carmel McCauley of the *Australian*, 'PAYE child maintenance plan'.

A few days later commentaries appeared. Kate Legge, re-porting on the reforms commented in the *Times on Sunday* on 5 April 1987: 'Hip pocket nerves have long been regarded as the most sensitive in the human body, but will they be pinched hard enough to curb the libido of partners who have no intention of sharing the cost of their offspring?'. Like many others, she came in behind the reforms but berated the gov-ernment for 'dithering' on the formula issue. The *Canberra Times* editorial on 31 March 1987, 'Justice for Parents', applau-ded the scheme and saw it as 'a more just system, even if one or two people suffer from a too-rigid application of the for-mula'. The *Age* editorial of the same date (p. 13), 'Defaulters pay at last', was similarly positive.

The other period of particular publicity about the reforms occurred in the first half of 1988, from around the time Parliament debated and then passed legislation enabling stage one of the scheme to occur, until the start-date of stage one on 1 June 1988. Ian Warden of the *Canberra Times* bemoaned the fact that the debate led to a 'bipartisan lull in the warfare between Government and Opposition since the Opposition has not had the nerve or the imagination to think of ways of opposing and criticising a piece of legislation which is designed to benefit children . . .' ('Concern for our greatest resource provides a lull in partisan warfare', 18 February 1988: 13). Deborah Stone, the *Australian*, reported on the reaction of the Lone Fathers Organisation, who were angry that the government refused to link its new legislation to access for NCPs ('"Non-access" may spark violence', 12 April 1988: 6) The next day

Kate Legge, *Melbourne Herald*, anticipated contents in the report of the CSCG on the formula ('Formula drawn up for child payments' 13 April 1988: 3). On 21 April in the *Age*, Mark Metherell placed the reforms in the context of assisting with 'the most intractable and unwanted result of what could be loosely described as the sexual revolution: child poverty' ('Scheme aims to cope with the legacy of sexual revolution', p. 13).

Once the report on formula was released, more press reaction followed; again not negative (e.g. Rod Campbell in the *Canberra Times*, 'Child maintenance "to fight poverty"', 11 May 1988: 3; Mark Metherell in the *Age* 'Separated parents may pay $98 weekly', 11 May 1988: 3; and Glenn Milne in the *Sydney Morning Herald*, 'Howe sets formula for divorce levy', 11 May 1988: 3.

head off criticism by sectional interests, to educate parents and employers about their rights and responsibilities, and to facilitate a smooth introduction and operation of the scheme.

EARLY DAYS OF DELIVERY

'The problem in implementing the more detailed aspects of policy was that there was no champion in the Tax Office. Further, they did not put on their brightest and best and therefore had people who "dragged their feet" . . . Internally the culture was ill-adapted to child support.' (Deena Shiff)

It is generally agreed by senior ATO officials that implementation by the ATO in the early days was poor. Tax officers were expected to undergo a major cultural shift in dealing face to face with clients, who were often distressed. When the Tax Commissioner, Trevor Boucher, served at the counter, he became acutely aware of the stress his staff were under and how untrained they were for the task. Tax officials claim that the original decisions and related resourcing did not take into account the need for this customer effort. Moreover, systems in operation were designed more for tax processes, for example batch processing rather than focusing activity on the counter. In any case, such a profound reform appended to existing Tax Office functions was bound to lead to early implementation problems.

Views from the Tax Office

'One thing that struck me was the stress on staff because they had to cope with emotional matters relating to the break-up of a

relationship, which was quite unrelated to the collection functions of CSA staff.' (Trevor Boucher)

'When I took over the CSA in 1994, people had no idea of what they were getting into. Women were ringing the ATO and effectively needing some form of marriage guidance counselling. This was not the ATO's understanding when it took over the Child Support Scheme. It was certainly not resourced to do that.' (Moira Scollay)

'The scheme had not won the hearts and minds of all of the senior people in the Tax Office; the folklore was that "we were told we had to have it". I was the eighth person in my position in four or five years, including people just before retirement. It was a time of downsizing and hence there was a chance to transfer staff into the agency. So we could have put more investment into the different skills and attitudes and qualities that people in child support would need and we did not put enough investment into that sort of thing . . . We also didn't anticipate enough the cultural shift required.' (David Butler)

'In the early days of setting up the scheme the caseload grew faster than expected, so the computer system could not cope. The management structure reflected that.' (Trevor Sutton)

EVALUATION

Stage 1 of the Child Support Scheme was subject to four major and publicly available evaluations between 1988 and 1991 (CSCG 1989, 1990; AIFS August 1990, June 1991). A major evaluation of both stages of the scheme also occurred in 1992 (CSEAG 1992). In addition, internal departmental evaluations took place. And in 1993 the scheme came under scrutiny by a Parliamentary Joint Select Committee.

Ministers and bureaucrats tussled over who should control the early evaluation process of Stage 1. Minister Howe was keen for the AIFS to be centrally involved; bureaucrats wanted as much say as possible. Howe gained support from his Cabinet colleagues to fund the AIFS, while bureaucrats succeeded in setting up a steering group for the AIFS evaluation, including departmental representatives. Former members of the CSCG were also members, which ensured continuity.

In August 1989 the CSCG reported on the operation of the scheme after fourteen months. It found, among other things, that there had been a substantial increase in coverage in terms of the number of children in sole-parent families receiving support: from 30 per cent of custodial parents receiving maintenance payments before the introduction of the scheme to between 60 and 70 per cent of custodial parents registered with the CSA and regularly receiving maintenance payments. In addition, it found that the average dollar amount of court orders had increased by 20–25 per cent under Stage 1. The report also drew attention to unsatisfactory features of the scheme, such as delays between making a court order and registering liability with the CSA and the arrears in collection.

In its final report on Stage 1 of the scheme, the evaluation group, now called the **Child Support Evaluation Advisory Group** (CSEAG), found that overall, the objectives set by the government were met. 'The[se] reforms seem, even in the relatively short time they have been in operation, to have been largely successful. The legislation, with some minor exceptions, appears to be working satisfactorily' (CSEAG 1990: iv).

At around the same time as the CSEAG first reported, the AIFS provided a preliminary report on a longitudinal study of the impact of Stage 1 (1990) followed by its final report in 1991, *Paying for the Children*. It saw the scheme moving collection and assessment of payments in the right direction, but with particular concerns about delays in payment to custodial parents.

The revenue clawback was not as high as expected but was sufficient in 1990 to offset administrative costs. Stage 2 was expected to make a much greater contribution.

The final evaluation report (1992) commented on the scheme as a whole. After noting the successes of the scheme in terms of more court orders and assessments and coverage of the scheme, it examined 'significant problems and deficiencies in the scheme', mainly in its administration (p. v). Complaints of NCPs who had second families were addressed as well as the need for simpler appeal processes and a recommendation (not acted on) for a retrospective scheme. The report saw it to be important to continue to monitor and refine the formula:

> The debate now is not whether child support should be assessed by a formula but whether the formula in Australia is satisfactory or whether it can be improved. The debate now is not whether child support obligations should be enforced through the Taxation Office but whether its procedures need to be improved so as to become more efficient and effective. A major effect of the scheme is a change in the community ethos so that support by parents is seen as a necessary consequence of their separation rather than as an exception. (CSEAG 1992, vol.1: iv)

Many refinements have been made to the scheme since 1992, with almost continuous evaluation and/or surveys of clients. While the broad policy framework appears robust, criticisms, especially from NCPs, continued to be directed towards the formula and administrative arrangements.

> 'Today we have more than a million parents using the Child Support Scheme and CSA; 44 per cent of those parents choose to transfer payments privately. Where the CSA is responsible for collection, it has collected 85 per cent of liabilities raised since the scheme's inception. So it has been successful in achieving policy outcomes . . . Before the scheme, less than 30 per cent of parents who had a court order for maintenance received payments. After ten years of operation, more than 70 per cent of parents are regularly paying child support, which is a fairly short period of time in the scheme of things.' (Catherine Argyll, letter to author, February 2000)

CONCLUSIONS

> 'While I regret a lot of child support history being eroded by time, the reality is that it is achieving the ultimate purpose . . . The purpose we set ourselves was to be in a position where, within a decade, social attitudes would have changed so that it would be a natural part of the scenery after people separated. That seems to be the position.' (John Fogarty)

> 'It was a remarkable feat to get up—such a controversial policy initiative and particularly one that had opposition from the public service.' (Derek Volker)

Few people believed in 1986 that the government would be able to introduce a scheme as radical as the proposal that the government committed itself to in the August 1987 Budget. Looking back to that period, it is also difficult to understand fully how such a radical social policy reform did come into being, especially given the complexity of the scheme and its sensitivity.

There were a number of serious obstacles to the Child Support Scheme getting off the ground:

- There were no models; no country had tried before to integrate an administrative and a court-based assessment system for collecting child maintenance.
- No country had yet delivered a collection and enforcement system based on the tax system.

- Bureaucratic resistance to the scheme was strong; no department wanted carriage of it (Edwards 1993); most officials were sceptical of such a radical reform succeeding and thought the government would see the error of its ways, right up to the passage of legislation.
- The policy crossed many portfolios, making it very difficult to drive any major policy reform, particularly when each agency has its own reasons for blocking reform.
- No lobby groups were pressing for radical reform; there was no momentum for change in a specific direction even though there was general recognition of the problem. In fact many lobby groups were suspicious of the motives of government, believing that its continued interest was revenue-driven. There was strong opposition to radical changes from the Law Council of Australia as well as from groups of NCPs.

In sum, the scheme looked as if it had little going for it. The opposing forces appeared too strong.

Why did the scheme see the light of day in the face of these obstacles? Many factors were at work and it is hard to sort out their relative importance. First, there was the determination of several Cabinet ministers for some reform, and their consequent close involvement in the development of the policy as well as the rather unusual processes they used to arrive at decisions. Brian Howe as the responsible minister was strategic in his use of processes. He also closely managed the parts of the bureaucracy that he could influence, including appointing his own consultant within his department and the use of the 'contacts' group of officials.

> *'The drive that came from the Minister himself—the fact that he was able to get the Treasurer, particularly, on side and the fact that it came in the broader context of major social security reform at a time when the integrity of the social security system was being supported and upheld.' (Derek Volker)*

Second, the child support reforms were placed in a broader policy context. This contrasts with the earlier attempt at reform in 1985, which had a focus on savings. The Child Support Scheme did have the attraction of savings (although not as large as originally expected), but the reforms were also intended to benefit sole-parent families, which meant there was harmony between the objectives of efficiency and equity.

Third, elements for successful problem identification were met: there was broad agreement on the nature of the problem; there was a prospect of a solution; it was an appropriate issue for government to put on the agenda; and it did not cut across the ideological position of the governing party (see Bridgman and Davis 1998: 36). This meant that stakeholders were ready to move on to examine possible approaches to reform.

Fourth, the policy analysis part of the process was rigorous and comprehensive. It was also more under the control of the Maintenance Secretariat and bureaucrats than other stages in the policy cycle. This case in particular demonstrates well how crucial it can be to ensure that key issues are identified and discussed by decision-makers before detailed work is undertaken on options. Discussions on key issues forced ministers to discuss principles to underlie the policy. This approach can bring to the fore issues of disagreement that require resolution. In the case of the Child Support Scheme, it was in fact more efficient at first to separate areas of disagreement from agreement and let the main framework for child support emerge from that process. In this case it was very important as a contribution to good policy outcomes to follow this approach.

Fifth, the child support policy was unusually complex for its day in the amount of coordination it required across departments, and the unusual processes used to achieve this, such as the formation of the Maintenance Secretariat.

'An important thing about child support was the good conceptual underpinning of the whole policy—there were very, very good people involved in both the Secretariat and the Minister's office; as well, people like Judge Fogarty were highly respected members of the community. There was a great deal of common sense and shrewdness involved in the whole process.' (Derek Volker)

Sixth, the effectiveness of the roles of and interactions between key players was another contributing factor to the success of the scheme. Much was also gained from the continuity of involvement of key people, for example Justice Fogarty, who was involved from the original conception of the idea through to evaluating the ultimate reforms. There was overlap of members of different bodies early in the problem definition and policy development stage, which brought some continuity of people over the period. Extremely useful connections existed, in particular between the Maintenance Secretariat staff and the legal profession, the Family Court, and welfare and women's organisations. In addition, secretariat staff made it their business and were adept (given their backgrounds outside the service) at being in constant touch with outside bodies to sound out their views, as well as the views of other departments. Many of the bureaucratic 'players' in the Maintenance Secretariat had a commitment, if not 'passion', for the reform. This led to a degree of tenacity not always found in public servants.

Other factors were the decision to implement the scheme in two stages when opposition to parts of it appeared insurmountable; the relative ineffectiveness of some hostile lobby groups, especially the Law Council of Australia; and the fact that enforcing access to children was addressed enough at the time of reform so that key NCP groups were, at least at that stage, satisfied.

It is interesting to ask the 'what if' questions. What if Brian Howe had not been the main player, but another minister, for example Senator Grimes? What if there had not been the interconnections of players on the FLC and the AIFS? What if the Law Council of Australia had been more effective in its lobby efforts? Could radical reform have been pursued with such vigour, and if so, succeeded? What if it had been the first and not the second Hawke government? The second Hawke government was looking for items to put on the agenda, whereas in its first term items for the agenda were created in advance.

So this is partly a timing issue. The external environment was right for introduction of this reform and reform was helped by having the right players on the scene at the right time.

> *'There seems to be a right time for reform. In this case: it would have been impossible to have generated the degree of support in the late 1970s or early 1980s but, as it turned out, this was a reform which came along at exactly the right moment. As you know, reforms do have their moment and if the opportunity is not then pressed, they can be lost.'* (John Fogarty, letter to author, July 1993)

A key lesson from this study is the need for those responsible for implementing policy to understand, if not agree with, the intentions of government, and hence to be closely involved in the policy development process. For example, with more goodwill between agencies, an expert group of DSS and ATO officials to examine effective systems could have been set up much earlier, to ease those problems at the start of the scheme. One of the failures of this exercise was that at no stage did the secretariat really understand the culture of the ATO. This was not for want of trying.

There are many ways in which the handling of the child support exercise could have been improved, although one can never determine the counterfactual. Certainly, to have had representatives of key departments operating from within the Maintenance Secretariat, as a team assisting the Cabinet Subcommittee, would have added more cohesion and effectiveness to the process.

HECS
CHRONOLOGY OF EVENTS 1985 TO AUGUST 1988

1985 Walsh proposes tertiary fees.

1986 HEAC introduced.

1987

July Dawkins appointed Minister for Employment, Education and Training.

September Dawkins issues paper, *The Challenge for Higher Education in Australia*.

November Membership and terms of reference of Wran Committee announced.

December Dawkins issued Green Paper, *Higher Education: A Policy Discussion Paper*.

1988

May Release of Report of Committee on Higher Education (Wran Report) and *The Wran Report: Commentary on Public Responses*.

June Tertiary charges debated at ALP Conference.

July Release of White Paper, *Higher Education; A Policy Statement*.

August Dawkins issues Budget statement *A New Commitment to Higher Education in Australia* in federal Budget context.

Four

Paying for a university education: HECS and not fees

The introduction of the Higher Education Contribution Scheme (HECS) in 1989 is one of the most successful policy formulations in Australia because it is both radical and enduring. In 1988, when the policy was developed, it was a radical change for the governing party that sponsored it (the ALP) because it seemed to repudiate a deep commitment of that party to free university education and was at first strongly opposed not only by students but also by other important constituencies of the ALP. The enduring character of HECS seems to have been confirmed recently (October 1999) when the present (Coalition) government hastily dropped an alleged proposal by the Minister for Education, Training and Youth Affairs, Dr Kemp, to abolish HECS and replace it by deregulated fees and an effective voucher system (Minister for Education and Youth Affairs, Media Release, Higher Education Funding, K10610, 18 October 1999).

By 1999 HECS had become an established feature of the higher education system in Australia, at least in the eyes of students, and the government recognised that changes to HECS could pose serious electoral hazards. The episode also demonstrated, indirectly, how radical changes to policies can fairly quickly become accepted as the normal state of affairs. When HECS was first introduced only ten years before, in 1989, it was viewed as a radical change from the previous system of university funding, and many saw it as a threat to the higher education aspirations of many students. It had some features that were new and untested in Australia and elsewhere.

The HECS that is currently operating is similar in principle, though different in some important details, to the scheme that was introduced ten years earlier. In essence, the HECS system gives students access to an interest-free loan to cover the fees they are charged at higher education institutions, with repayments contingent on their income being above a threshold level. Annual repayments of the loans, indexed to inflation, are directly deducted by the Australian Tax Office. The deferred payment scheme is supplemented by an option for students to pay the contribution upfront at a discounted rate.

Since HECS was first introduced, the scheme has become much less generous from the students' perspective: annual student fees have been substantially increased (from a standard fee of $1800 in 1989 to fees in the range $3409–5682, dependent mainly on the costs of courses); rates of repayment have been at least doubled (from 1 per cent of income in 1989 to 3 per cent in 1999 for those in lower income brackets, and from 3 per cent of income in 1989 to 6 per cent in 1999 for those in higher income brackets); and the thresholds at which repayments of loans begin have been reduced.

HISTORY AND CONTEXT

In 1974 ALP Prime Minister Gough Whitlam abolished fees for higher education in Australia. Free education was a core element of the Labor platform. Fees paid at the time of tuition ('upfront' fees) were considered inequitable and a barrier to access by poorer members of society. Thus their abolition was an ideological policy decision of the new ALP Government and remains one of the most remembered actions of that government.

It was not long before the issue of fees returned to the political agenda, as student numbers increased, funds for universities became scarcer, and reintroduction of some fees began to seem inevitable. Soon after the Fraser Government came to power in 1975, there was discussion within the Coalition parties about reintroducing fees, but it was not until 1981 that a significant step in this direction was taken with the introduction of fees for second and higher-degree students. This was despite a commitment given by the Fraser Government during the 1980 federal election campaign that it would not reintroduce fees (Hansard, HR, 21 October 1981: 2323).

In 1985, under the Hawke Labor Government, the Minister for

Finance, Peter Walsh, proposed reintroducing some form of charge on tertiary students. He strongly advocated the introduction of an income-tested, fee-based system, believing that this was the most effective way of raising revenue from within the sector from those most able to pay. Such a scheme was, however, politically infeasible within the ALP, and Walsh found little support.

As an alternative, the Higher Education Administrative Charge (HEAC) was introduced in 1986. The HEAC was an annual fee paid by all tertiary students and set initially at a rate of $250 per annum to cover the university's per student administration costs.

> The 'administrative charge' was a substitute for tertiary fees, but was approximately equal to the administration—as distinct from tuition, capital and maintenance—cost in universities. Two years later it was replaced by the Higher Education Contribution Scheme (HECS). Both schemes are inferior, fiscally and administratively, to the income-tested fee proposed in 1985. (Walsh 1995: 152)

There was a policy weakness in HEAC: it could not raise sufficient revenue to fund any significant expansion of the higher education sector. Institutions retained only 10 per cent of revenue raised, and growth in income from this source was tied to student numbers (Dawkins 1987b: 84). As well, there was opposition to HEAC on equity grounds, making it unpopular within the ALP and among the community. The equity impact of HEAC was demonstrated after its first year of operation when enrolment figures for 1987 showed a fall in the numbers of female and part-time students entering university (Power and Robertson 1987).

THE EXTERNAL ENVIRONMENT

HECS was a product of the 1980s, during which growing student numbers, a government concerned about ensuring access to education by disadvantaged groups, and increasing constraints on government spending forced universities and government to look for new ways of providing higher education. HECS was also a product of a political party—the ALP—that had a special commitment to higher education and was in government for most of the 1980s. And it was a product of a period in which new approaches to public management were emerging, approaches that placed high emphasis on 'performance' and 'efficiency' in the provision of public services (even though HECS, as it turned out, was more about equity than efficiency). There were comparisons of the performance of Australian universities with those in other countries, and heightened interest in how universities might contribute to improving Australia's economic performance and international competitiveness. These points are elaborated below.

The growth in student numbers from the mid-1970s was dramatic. The total number of students enrolled in higher education increased by about 42 per cent. Despite this, it was estimated that in 1987 up to 20 000 qualified applicants were unable to obtain places in higher education. It was evident, furthermore, that future growth in numbers of university students would also have to be substantial if, to meet government objectives, a higher proportion of school students were to have the opportunity of continuing their education at tertiary level, and more graduates were to be produced.

Second, there was an increasing shortage of federal funding for higher education. Reflecting the desire of the government to be a 'low-tax country', and hence wanting a tighter budgetary situation, the funds provided by the Commonwealth Government each year for higher education during this period had remained around $2.5 billion. As GDP had been growing, spending on higher education represented a declining proportion of GDP, from 1.4 per cent in 1975 to 1 per cent in 1987; and as student numbers had been sharply increasing over the period, funds per student had dropped by 23 per cent.

Projections made in 1987 of desirable student numbers up to 2001 pointed to funding requirements in 2001 that were from 30 to 40 per cent above expenditure planned in the 1987/88 Budget. This shortfall made no allowance for a 'heavy backlog of capital and equipment' or for 'any additional funds required to achieve improvements in the quality of education' (Dawkins 1987: 79, 124, 126). In short, in 1987 the combination of growing student numbers and severe shortages of funds pointed to an impending crisis in higher education.

Third, was the commitment of the ALP to improving access to higher education. This was partly reflected in targets for a rising student population, mentioned above, and partly in the ALP's 1986 platform as an important equity measure. Like its predecessors over many years, this platform included a commitment to 'maintain the provision of free tertiary education,' which had begun with the Whitlam Government's abolition of university fees in 1974. This commitment meant there were serious ideological barriers to introducing student fees.

Fourth, was the emerging managerialist approach in public administration, which in the field of higher education prompted consideration of the goals and performance of universities, in terms of 'outcomes' and 'outputs', and the 'efficiency' with which these were achieved. One effect of this was to encourage comparisons of the performance of Australian universities with those in other countries, and to give prominence to findings of an OECD study that rated Australia fairly poorly in its output of graduates per head of population (e.g. see CTEC 1987).

A related effect was to encourage consideration of how universities could contribute to improving Australia's economic performance and international competitiveness by enhancing skill levels in the population and also by 'exporting' higher education to other countries, through programs for overseas students.

Thus many factors were at work that placed importance on increasing the number of graduates in the population. In particular, the managerialist approach encouraged consideration of different ways of funding higher education, such as through user-pays arrangements rather than taxes. It encouraged reflection on the results of research showing that the introduction of free university education in 1974 had failed to produce the revolution in access to higher education that had been expected (Anderson and Vervoorn 1983: 171).

ENTER DAWKINS

The immediate context for the development of what became HECS was the federal election of July 1987, following which John Dawkins was appointed Minister for Employment, Education and Training. One of his colleagues has described Dawkins as 'a man whose zeal and ambition for change were yoked to an abrasive and pugnacious approach that added to the turbulence that swirled around him. A moody, self-contained figure, contemptuous of both the foolish and the spineless, he was little loved in the caucus or even in his own centre-left faction, surviving on his talents alone' (Blewett 1999: 16).

Dawkins had been shadow minister for education between November 1980 and January 1983. After the ALP came to power in March 1983, he was appointed Minister for Finance (March 1983 to December 1984) and after that Minister for Trade (December 1984 to July 1987). Thus when he gained responsibility for education policy in July 1987, he brought to the task not only a reforming zeal and knowledge of education issues from his days as shadow minister, but also a familiarity with budgetary issues and a commitment to managerial approaches in public administration from his period as Minister for Finance, as well as a perspective on the potential contribution of higher education to international competitiveness from his period as Minister for Trade. It might be noted that the ministry to which Dawkins was appointed—Employment, Education and Training—brought the functions of employment and education under one portfolio for the first time in the history of Australian federal government, to emphasise the links the government wanted to make between education and national economic objectives.

> *'Dawkins saw higher education as an export commodity, tied to the question of trade. He believed higher education needed to be more robust if it was to stand up to international competition. Plus he believed it had to become a more utilitarian sector, linked more directly to the needs of industry.' (Mike Gallagher)*

STRUCTURES AND PLAYERS

> One of the problems for economists who are directly involved in policy-making is that the standard textbooks tell us close to nothing about process. However, successfully managing issues of process is critical to policy change. Indeed, no matter how correct are the ideas, how well researched are the likely impacts, and how on-side are the major direct political players, without the endorsement and support of the bureaucracy significant advances are unlikely. (Chapman 1996a: 12)

Of utmost importance to the acceptance and success of HECS was the organisational process that occurred during the policy's formulation. This process made possible the radical policy shift that HECS represented as well as facilitating its later acceptance within the ALP and the broader community.

The organisational process involved several key steps. First, a taskforce of officials was established to review all aspects of higher education in Australia and to draft the Green Paper on higher education (Dawkins 1987b). Second, the Wran Committee was convened specifically to investigate higher education funding. This was followed, after the ALP Conference in June, by a White Paper, *Higher Education: A Policy Statement* (Dawkins 1988a), published in July 1988 before Dawkins issued his paper 'A New Commitment to Higher Education in Australia' as a budget statement, including the announcement of HECS a month later (1988b).

Closely associated with decisions Dawkins made on organisational processes and important to HECS's eventual success was the selection of key individuals for their particular backgrounds and skills to work either on the taskforce or as members of the Wran Committee or its secretariat. What follows elaborates on the Green Paper and Wran Committee processes.

The Green Paper Taskforce

Shortly before the formation of this taskforce, the government merged two federal departments to create the Department of Employment,

Education and Training (DEET). This merger was significant. It highlighted the new philosophy Dawkins sought for higher education in Australia, one that linked higher education directly to employment, making it more responsive and reactive to the needs of the labour market. It also caused considerable disruption and turmoil in the affected parts of the federal public service.

Dawkins drew the taskforce's staff from this new Commonwealth department. But he deliberately employed those who came from its employment and training, rather than education, divisions. In this way he selected staff who appreciated the needs of the labour market and whose thinking was unlikely to be restricted by existing policy practices, most notably those associated with the Commonwealth Tertiary Education Commission. He chose people who he believed were capable of formulating and implementing radical change in Australian higher education.

In what was soon to prove a most beneficial move, an ANU economist, Bruce Chapman, was appointed as a full-time consultant to Dawkins' department to assist with the Green Paper but went on to play a crucial role within the taskforce assisting the Wran Committee.

The Wran Committee and its secretariat

The Green Paper announced that the government would establish a committee to examine 'possible options in this area', and provide recommendations by February–March 1988. The paper ended with what became, without amendment, the terms of reference for the second and major analytical report, by the Wran Committee, on funding issues. The committee's terms of reference were devised by Bruce Chapman and David Phillips.

Recognising that radical changes to the system of student fees would be controversial within the community as well as in his own party, Dawkins appointed members to the committee who were strategically chosen because of their high standing professionally and among those who would have to be persuaded; and because he believed these people were capable of generating innovative policy. The chair was Neville Wran, a former premier of NSW and a highly respected political figure within and beyond the ALP, whose status and authority would later be of great importance in gaining support for the committee's recommendations, especially from the NSW Labor Right.

A second member of the committee was Meredith Edwards, a senior public servant then in the Department of Social Security, who had strong academic qualifications and experience with student issues from her involvement in the development of AUSTUDY. She also

---

The Wran Committee terms of reference

The government is committed to expanding the capacity and effectiveness of the higher education sector and to improving access to higher education for groups that are currently under-represented. This goal has significant funding implications, as outlined in the Policy Discussion Paper on higher education. Given current and likely future budgetary circumstances, the government believes that it is necessary to consider sources of funding involving the direct beneficiaries of higher education.

The committee should develop options and make recommendations for possible schemes of funding which could involve contributions from higher education students, graduates, their parents and employers. In developing options, the committee should have regard to the social and educational consequences of the schemes under examination. (Dawkins 1987b: 87)

---

had experience in the development of policies on child support, which was significant in negotiating the assistance of the Taxation Office in collecting payments from individuals for the later administration of HECS.

The third member was Bob Gregory, a highly regarded economist from the ANU, who had extensive experience in providing policy advice to governments and in research relevant to the work of the committee.

The secretary of the committee was Mike Gallagher, also a senior public servant, then in charge of the Office of Local Government in the Department of Immigration, Local Government and Ethnic Affairs, who had considerable experience in education policy and university politics. He was known to Dawkins, who trusted him to provide a professional service to the Wran Committee outside the established bureaucracy.

> 'Dawkins was very calculating in who he had working on the committee. He needed above all political consensus within the ALP at the end—especially because HECS was such a radical shift from the ALP Platform.' (Mike Gallagher)

The secretariat that produced the Wran paper, as with the Green Paper, was picked from Dawkins' department, but mostly from areas outside higher education. Significantly, many of its members had also been part of the Green Paper Taskforce. This helped the committee to progress quickly from the position reached by the taskforce, politically as well as analytically. That is, views presented in the taskforce report could be expected to pervade material prepared for the committee, and analysis undertaken for the taskforce could be readily used by and further developed for the committee.

> 'A deliberate decision was taken to draw people onto the secretariat of the Wran Committee from across other areas of the newly formed Department of Employment, Education and Training. There was a view that the Higher Education Division of the former Commonwealth Department of Education might be too linked to the current approach.' (Chris Robinson)

Dawkins kept in close touch with the work of the Wran Committee through David Phillips, a member of his staff who had worked with Edwards on youth allowance reform (Chapter 2). He attended all meetings of the committee as observer and as 'the Minister's eyes and ears'; he kept in contact also with members of the committee's secretariat. Further in the background was Paul Hickey, then head of the Higher Education Division in DEET, to whom Alison Weeks, the secretariat's director, reported regularly and who, apparently, 'read every draft' (Weeks, interview).

Dawkins had Treasurer Paul Keating on side. Keating approached Trevor Boucher, head of the ATO at the time, and said: 'I am not sure what scheme Dawkins is developing but he is one of the few with new ideas, so support him if you can' (Boucher, interview).

Alongside the above, Dawkins used the education subcommittee of Caucus most strategically and kept it informed of relevant materials; when it was divided on the issues, he made sure the subcommittee did not put those issues to the vote, since that could have counted against the cause at the forthcoming ALP conference.

Dawkins' concern to establish an independent but sympathetic secretariat to undertake the policy analysis for changes in higher education illustrates a problem that is not uncommon in policy-making generally, namely how to achieve the 'right' result without compromising the quality and integrity of the analysis. From the perspective of a reforming minister, radical change could typically be expected to encounter bureaucratic resistance, and establishment of a secretariat that understood the broader context would be one way of working around this resistance. The organisation and staffing of policy analysis activities is thus often a very important aspect of policy-making, particularly when radical changes are envisaged.

IDENTIFYING THE ISSUES

By July 1987, when Dawkins was given ministerial responsibility for higher education, the issue of charging university fees had been on

THE PLAYERS

Ministers

Dawkins, John	Minister for Employment, Education and Training
Keating, Paul	Treasurer
Walsh, Peter	Minister for Finance

Wran Committee members

Edwards, Dr Meredith	Member, Head of Social Policy Division, DSS
Gallagher, Mike	Committee Secretary, Head of Office of Local Government
Gregory, Prof. Bob	Member, Professor of Economics, ANU
Wran, Neville	Committee Chair, ex–Premier of New South Wales

Secretariat

The Secretariat consisted of a small group of people drawn from DEET with Alison Weeks, Director (and previously Head of the Green Paper Taskforce). It also included Chris Robinson and Dr Bruce Chapman, departmental consultant, an economist from the ANU.

Public servants

Boucher, Trevor	Tax Commissioner, ATO
Grant, Peter	Assistant Secretary, Higher Education Division, DEET, 1985
Hickey, Paul	Head, Higher Education Division, DEET
Podger, Andrew	Division Head, Department of Finance
Rose, Dennis	Principal adviser, AGs Department

Other

Aitkin, Prof. Don	Chair, Australian Research Committee
Davidson, Ken	Journalist, the *Age*
Evans, Kiri	President of National Students' Association
Mawer, Allen	Senior adviser to Minister for Employment, Education and Training
Milne, Dr Frank	Academic, ANU
Phillips, David	Senior adviser to Minister for Employment, Education and Training
Stretton, Prof. Hugh	University of Adelaide

the political agenda intermittently for over ten years, and therefore the particular issues that were starting to emerge were not so much whether but when fees should be introduced and what form they should take. It had become evident to Dawkins by then that a fundamental review of higher education and its funding was essential, and at the policy stage of 'identifying the Issues' this meant identifying those features of the environment that were seen to be driving change, and the broad questions that should be addressed.

PUTTING THE PROBLEM ON THE AGENDA

Dawkins released a brief paper in September 1987 titled *The Challenge for Higher Education in Australia*. This paper signalled the government's intention to develop 'a new set of arrangements for Commonwealth support of higher education from the beginning of 1989' (Dawkins 1987a: 3). It attempted to set the scene for a public debate on the future of higher education in Australia, and announced the establishment of a taskforce of officials from Dawkins' department to 'confront the range of concerns the Government holds about the current performance of our higher education system' (p. 10).

The first part of the paper provided an overview of the higher education system, giving the government's assessment of the environment and key issues for policy-making. It referred to the 'demographic bulge in the youth age group', which had created an 'unprecedented demand for higher education places' (p. 6), and noted that in the current budgetary and economic circumstances it was 'simply not feasible to achieve quantum leaps in participation in higher education by providing quantum leaps in public expenditure' (p. 7). It stated that Australia lagged behind its international competitors 'on a range of significant measures of education and training performance, including . . . the level of youth participation in higher education, and the proportion of the workforce holding post-school qualifications' (p. 5). In words that have gained significance with hindsight, the paper stated that it would be necessary for 'the [university] institutions themselves, State Governments, the private sector, staff and students' to address such problems, together with the government.

The paper included a qualified invitation to universities to examine alternatives to government funding, described somewhat elliptically as a 'means of enabling institutions to increase revenue from private sources and hence their ability to deliver services, bearing in mind the Australian Labor Party's policy of opposition to tuition fees' (p. 12).

Dawkins' paper thus set a broad framework and tone for the sweeping review of higher education that he envisaged. He believed

that a significant expansion in higher education was a fundamental
precondition for Australia's economic success, but he also thought it
unfair to expect taxpayers to fund all of the growth in places that
were needed. Unlike Walsh's earlier aborted attempt at reintroducing
fees, Dawkins had identified the problem differently and set an
all-encompassing context without actually canvassing the reintroduction of fees. The taskforce of carefully selected officials produced a
document for Dawkins which heralded that review and was published
as the Green Paper *Higher Education: A Policy Discussion Paper* in
December 1987 (Dawkins 1987b).

THE ROLE OF THE GREEN PAPER

Although the Green Paper was described as a 'discussion paper', it
was clear that Dawkins was looking to it to provide a basis for the
radical changes he saw as necessary in the higher education system.
Thus in his foreword he noted that 'The issues [the paper] raises,
and the policy responses to which it leads, will have a vital influence
on the directions of higher education development in Australia
through to the turn of the century' (Dawkins 1987b: iv).

The general style of the paper was strongly polemical, with more
statements of government intentions than explorations of options.

The Green Paper was essentially an elaboration of the increasingly difficult environment confronting higher education, leading to
the broad conclusion that radical change was inevitable. The first
part, 'Assessing the challenge', addressed the issues outlined on
pp. 99–101 above, and it concluded with an affirmation of the
government's intention to improve access to higher education. The
second part, 'A unified national system', addressed structural and
management issues in higher education, and foreshadowed further
major institutional changes. The third part, 'Funding the system',
elaborated on the increasing funding constraints for higher education
and the emerging 'funding gap' (Dawkins 1987b: 81).

The paper proposed 'far-reaching reforms in organisation and
practice of higher education' (Dawkins 1987b: 1). The key changes
included:

- the creation of a unified national higher education system
- the rationalisation of higher education institutions around the
  country
- altered advisory arrangements, including the establishment of
  the National Board of Employment, Education and Training
  (NBEET), the Higher Education Council (HEC) and the Australian Research Council (ARC)

- new funding arrangements whereby universities received triennial funding via single operating grants from which institutions were free to decide spending priorities.

These reforms were to 'provide the basis for a long-term expansion of the higher education system and greater access to the system and its benefits' (Dawkins 1988b: 2).

In the restrained and bland way that official reports can hint of major changes and provide a lead-in to the next stage of policy analysis, the discussion paper concluded with some comments on 'other funding options'. After noting that there was 'considerable scope for institutions to raise additional revenue from non-Commonwealth sources', it stated: 'One additional source of funds that may need to be considered is a contribution from individual students, former students and/or their parents'. It alluded briefly to what was seen as, and would become in later public debate, a major argument for reintroducing student fees, namely 'that graduates of higher education experience, on average, highly favourable labour market outcomes compared with those without tertiary qualifications'. Strategically omitting funding policy options for discussion, it commented that the issues 'are much more complex than this, given that private contribution schemes would have implications for, among other things, equity, access and the overall level and composition of the student body'. It went on:

> In the present and likely future budgetary climate, constraints on funding to the higher education sector are expected to continue. It is difficult for the Commonwealth alone to provide for significant expansion in higher education enrolments, despite the benefits—economic and otherwise—that will result. Additional sources of funding will need to be investigated, having regard to both the public and private benefits that higher education confers. (Dawkins 1987b: 75)

The Green Paper was originally going to include a chapter devoted to options for financing higher education. Dawkins had commissioned his consultant Bruce Chapman to write that chapter. The drafted chapter identified the nature of the problem but also included options for financing, such as upfront fees with scholarships (at the time apparently favoured by Dawkins) as well as a proposal preferred by Chapman and others in Dawkins' office (especially Allen Mawer) and similar to HECS. Once Dawkins read this material, it was clear to him that the complexities and sensitivities of financing issues, especially fees, meant that these issues had to be handled separately rather than addressed in the Green Paper.

'When the ERC was looking for savings and revenue in 1985, Dawkins' office was casting about for ideas that would be less

politically damaging in policy and party terms than some of the things, like HEAC, that were in contemplation. In the event we came up empty and the students got HEAC, but in December 1995 you sent me a copy of the child support paper you, Harper and Harrison had prepared for the Law and Society Conference. I was taken with the creative use of the tax system to recover state outlays . . .

'What Dawkins was really looking for was a painless way to introduce fees. You will recall that when he knew the answer and only expected you to find a way of getting him to it, the trick was to find an opportunity to intrude a lateral thought. That occurred when he was talking in his office one day to Don Aitkin, mainly about the ARC, but also about higher education. I was the mandatory staffer present. Dawkins was again musing about where the money could come from so I suggested, in about the 30 seconds I reckoned I could hold his attention, that

- *students could repay after graduation through the tax system*
- *the repayment regime could be tailored to the aggregate contribution required by government—at its most extreme, if all graduates paid, whether they benefitted or not, for the whole of their working lives, in theory the higher education system could eventually be made to support itself*
- *the main argument of the 'no-fees' element in the party— restriction of access—would fall to the ground.*

'Put as baldly as this, and I confess that my own thinking had not gone much further, it was a graduate tax, not an income-contingent loan repayment scheme for all students, but the approach registered with Dawkins.' (Allen Mawer, letter to author, 7 February 2000)

The obvious place to begin to seek the needed revenue was students—the most readily identifiable beneficiaries of the sector. Two main arguments were used by Dawkins to justify charging students directly: that students received private benefits from higher education; and that higher education post-Whitlam was not 'free', but rather a form of 'middle-class welfare'.

PRIVATE AND PUBLIC BENEFITS OF HIGHER EDUCATION

Much evidence was available that suggested that students receive personal benefits from participation in tertiary education. Income and employment rates provide the most obvious indicators of this private benefit: 'Lifetime incomes are typically much higher, unemployment rates are lower and the expected duration of unemployment is relatively short for those with university degrees' (Chapman 1998: 121).

While these statistics imply a private benefit to the individual from participation in higher education, this is not the only form of benefit identifiable. There is also considerable public benefit from having an educated community. The positive spillover effects include·

- political and social benefits from better informed public debate and voting behaviour
- community benefits from research and technological developments
- the transferral of skills to those who have not received a tertiary education
- economic benefits to the broader community, including greater growth potential, higher wages and, consequently, tax revenue, increased attractiveness to investment and a more adaptable workforce (Chapman 1997: 8).

Taken together, these numerous public benefits suggest that there is considerable social value in having an educated group in the community; they also provide a strong justification for some level of government funding of higher education to ensure that these public benefits are maximised.

While the existence of private benefits implies that individuals should pay something towards the cost of their tertiary education, the existence of public benefits implies that the amount paid by students should be only a proportion of that cost.

'FREE' HIGHER EDUCATION IS 'MIDDLE-CLASS WELFARE'

The second and powerful argument used to justify charging students was that 'free' higher education was in reality 'middle-class welfare', to which all taxpayers contributed but from which the better-off mostly benefited; since 1974, students had not paid to attend university, making higher education free of charge. However, the higher education sector ran at considerable cost. This cost was met almost entirely by the Federal Government from its general tax revenue, which was obtained from all taxpayers, despite the majority of Australian taxpayers having never participated in or benefited personally from the universities they were funding.

Not only had they not benefited personally, but the majority of Australian taxpayers were, on average, less well off than those they were supporting through the provision of 'free' tertiary education. As mentioned previously, the demographic breakdown of the student population revealed that most students came from relatively well-off socioeconomic backgrounds. Further, students, on average, became relatively better-off following their education. This argument was crucial in selling the need for change.

Focusing on the inequity of the current funding arrangements opened the way for considering the reintroduction of fees because it highlighted flaws in the original argument used to justify their abolition. This articulation of the policy problem claimed that higher education, while free to students, was at significant cost to taxpayers. The argument naturally led on to the question of how this cost could be met. That was to be the issue of concern. Highlighting the inequity and regressivity of 'free' higher education in this way proved later to be vitally important in selling the problem and in convincing the ALP, the tertiary sector and others of the merits of HECS.

In 1987, therefore, the policy issue was clearly identified: increased revenue was required to expand Australia's higher education sector in order to meet greater demand for university places, especially at a time of straitened government funds. Further, this revenue had to be raised from those groups who benefited directly from the higher education sector, most notably students because they were the most easily identifiable beneficiaries. The revenue had to be raised in such a way that it did not deter access. The problem posed to the Wran Committee was therefore a well-structured policy problem, articulated in economic efficiency terms but with a heavy emphasis on equity benefits.

POLICY ANALYSIS

The nature of the policy analysis undertaken on higher education funding was broadly shaped by the vision Dawkins had for radical change in the system, and his perceptions of the resistance that might be encountered to such change. While he wanted analysis of the big issues in higher education to be broadly supportive of his vision, he also realised the importance of having rigorous arguments for specific proposals that would stand up to scrutiny by the interest groups most likely to be critical of change.

Most of the analysis on higher education charging and the related package of measures was undertaken in the context of the secretariat that Dawkins set up to support the Wran team. All this was undertaken within a year of Dawkins' appointment to the position of Minister for Employment, Education and Training in July 1987.

In late 1987 the **Wran Committee**, or **Committee on Higher Education Funding** as it was officially known, was convened with the specific purpose of developing options for deriving a contribution from those who benefit directly from participating in higher education. Furthermore, this contribution had to be equitable and efficient and improve access to higher education by under-represented groups. The *Report of the Committee on Higher Education Funding* (the Wran Report) was published in May 1988 and distributed for public comment.

DATA AND RESEARCH

New as it was in Australian policy formulation, the idea of levying graduates after they were in receipt of income is not a new concept. It can be traced back to the well-known economist Milton Friedman (1955). Before the period of this particular case study, several people had written about one or another form of a graduate levy or tax (e.g. Blandy 1979; Barr 1987; Bulbeck 1987; Manning 1986; Wells 1987). What was radical was that Dawkins picked up an academic idea and ran with it as a policy.

Dr Bruce Chapman played a pivotal role in using formal economic tools to advantage and in providing important economic data and research to the Wran Committee as well as to Dawkins. For example, he unearthed evidence to show convincingly that, for Australia, on average, higher education is associated with private economic returns, which strongly made a case for charging (Chapman 1996a: 4).

As further evidence, several studies in the mid-1980s revealed that despite the abolition of fees from 1974, the socioeconomic composition of undergraduate students attending university had changed little since Whitlam's historic decision. Especially influential in affecting attitudes to reform was the work of Anderson and Vervoorn:

> The problem of crude measures was highlighted in the recent discussion over the effects of fee abolition from 1974. Analysis of the social composition of the student body before and after the change revealed no discernible difference in the social spectrum of higher education. Nevertheless this does not permit the conclusion that the removal of fees did not enable poor students to enrol who otherwise would have been deterred; if there were such students—and common sense suggests that there must have been—either they were not sufficiently numerous to show up in statistical aggregates, or their poverty was not revealed by the questions directed at parental status etc. (1983: 172)

The Green Paper Taskforce, carefully collected data, and research results such as the above were to provide evidence for the Wran Committee on the socioeconomic status of students. They made much of the point that there had been little change since fees were abolished in 1974, as outlined in the Wran Report.

An important issue for the broader community was whether the introduction of charges for higher education would reduce the demand for places. It was politically important to provide evidence to convince sceptics that the financing outcome would be equitable and would not make the socioeconomic composition at universities worse: the secretariat and Chapman were rigorous in gathering relevant data and research on this issue which showed that, for both sexes, the rates of return to investment in higher education remained high after the imposition of a charge:

> It is of policy interest that the facts concerning where higher educa-
> tion students come from in socio-economic terms, and where they
> end up in terms of relative earnings, were not questioned by the polit-
> ical opponents of the introduction of a charge. This was important to
> the eventual commitment of the Labor Government to the policy.
> (Chapman 1996a: 6)

Evidence was also scanned for the impact of the HEAC. As the Wran Report indicated, tentative evidence was that part-time and mature-age students, especially women, appeared to have been deterred; and researchers Power and Robertson (1987) had concluded similarly.

These few examples of where data and research were gathered and undertaken help to refine the problem at hand and to clarify issues. Without the rigour behind this stage in policy analysis and the reassurance, especially about equity aspects of the proposed reform, key stakeholders may well have been in a position to thwart that reform.

The Wran Committee gave much attention to overseas experience in the funding of higher education: a chapter of its report was devoted to summarising practices in several countries. Higher education institutions in many other countries were, like those in Australia, experiencing problems from increasing student numbers and decreasing government funds, and were searching for alternative ways of funding higher education. Reflecting this, the OECD had produced several studies on these issues, to which Dawkins had referred in his preface to the Green Paper. While consideration of practices in other countries can be a source of new ideas in policy analysis, international comparisons can also help to strengthen arguments for positions already reached. This was largely the case with HECS, because of novel features that went beyond overseas practices. The reporting on overseas practices was assisted by an overseas trip by Alison Weeks. She returned with an important piece of information about the high rate of default on loans where they were provided through the banking system in other countries.

KEY ISSUES FOR THE WRAN COMMITTEE

The objectives of this committee were quite clear: they were stated in the terms of reference and had been subsequently added to by the Minister when he declared, in a public statement, that 'equity issues were paramount'.

What 'equity' actually meant became an issue for the committee. Perhaps the most important issue of all to emerge was what assumptions were to be made about financial dependence of students on their parents, or in the case of the mature-aged, on their partners. One view was that the family could be assumed to support students and so, from an equity viewpoint, it should not be of concern if higher-income families had to pay fees upfront. The key inequity from this perspective was that the well off (or middle class) could afford to pay for their children to go to university, and that this should not be a burden on lower-income taxpayers. This line of argument led to viewing fees (possibly with loans) and scholarships based on a family income test as an equitable option.

> 'I remember Neville Wran describing free education as people in [Sydney's] western suburbs paying tax so that the children of parents on the North Shore could send their children to university for free.' (Mike Gallagher)

The other perspective was that such a regime could disadvantage students who were not able to share in family income, for whatever reason. There was some evidence that this could be more of a problem for women than for men, and particularly for women in non-metropolitan areas where, from a past era, teacher's scholarships had been so beneficial for their participation in education. According to this line of argument, any charge for tuition would need to be levied on individual income, according to capacity to pay.

A related and broader issue was the extent to which the need for revenue should be traded off against equity: if there were to be some form of charge contingent on income, then the revenue flow would be less than if upfront fees were introduced.

Certain other issues needed careful debate but moved more easily to consensus:

- the extent to which a public subsidy should be provided given no clear evidence on what proportion of total cost led to public benefit (discussed below)
- whether to index the debt only to inflation or to include a real rate of interest (resolved in favour of the former on equity grounds)
- where to set the income thresholds

- how the charge should relate to the cost of a course.

For the third meeting of the Wran Committee in January 1988, Alison Weeks provided an overview document intended to serve as a starting point for detailed analysis of these issues and consequent options. In a well-structured approach, the document listed some key issues requiring early resolution, one of those issues being what weighting the committee wanted to give the criteria by which those options would be chosen.

The Wran Committee did not move unhesitatingly to its preferred position on an income-contingent loans scheme. The differences within the committee on the relative merits of means-tested upfront fees for students and deferred, income-contingent payment of fees by graduates continued over several meetings. Dawkins too was initially doubtful about the latter approach. The issue was partially resolved, as such issues commonly are, at the culmination of a long and painstaking process of policy analysis, in the setting of an informal and convivial dinner attended by the members of the committee and the secretariat. But whether there should still be an upfront fee on students in the highest (e.g. 20 per cent) of families rather than a discount for payment upfront, continued as a dividing issue. While the Wran Committee was debating these issues, the debate was also occurring outside government, for example:

> There is solid support building in the ALP Caucus, academia and the Department of Employment, Education and Training for the imposition of a tax on the incomes of university graduates as an alternative to reintroducing tertiary education fees. (*AFR*, 23 February 1988: 1)

In early March the views of academics were prominent in the press. The *Australian* (2 March 1988) published a page on the graduate tax debate where the views of two academics, who favoured both the Wran proposals and a graduate tax or levy, were aired in journalist's articles: Professor Murray Wells, then head of Sydney University Economics Faculty (article by William West), and Roger Eade, Footscray Institute of Technology, on the benefits of a graduate levy, based on his submission to the Wran Committee (article by Christopher Dawson). About this time there was also a leak to the press of a Department of Finance position paper on funding of higher education.

DEVELOPING OPTIONS

Frustrations of a player

7 March 1988 I rang Bob Gregory just to keep in touch to be told about a Finance submission to us (which I hadn't received) which had been leaked to the press. Gregory apparently had suggested to Finance, having seen it earlier, that it be sent to us. It wasn't even marked 'Cabinet-in-Confidence'! A lot of press this week on education funding, which has been making me a bit nervous plus my worry that ATO would walk away from the proposal.

13 March 1988 Up at 6 a.m. Saturday to read most of first draft of Higher Education charging report. Disturbed by realisation that we cannot only recommend a levy on exit because effectively there would be no revenue for a couple of years. Rang Bruce to talk about discounting upfront compared to a compulsory levy on rich parents.

I enjoyed Monday: visit to Sydney to meet with Wran and Gregory et al. Turned around the meeting yet again . . . I feel every time I work very hard to do that. Mike Gallagher was very helpful.

21 March 1988 Wednesday—all morning taken up with DEET's higher education charging issues. I felt drained at the end of it as I felt so much was at stake as I was being pressured to accept a compulsory upfront charge on students with rich parents.

27 March 1988 All afternoon with Higher Education taskforce and exhausted myself arguing hard against the viewpoint of a bright but obstinate member of the secretariat on wanting upfront fees for the top 20 per cent. Angry at having my time wasted. Bruce Chapman suggested that Bob G. and Mike G. and I meet on our own to sort out a position, which we did on Thursday, and that worked well. They agreed to leave revenue-raising options open knowing I would deliver a minority statement otherwise.

17 April 1988 Wran Committee went well but exhausting and fought over how high the threshold level of income should be rather than how to get the quick buck. Apparently in the half-hour after I left (and before Wran left), the Committee backtracked on where I was at. But fortunately the report as I saw it this weekend has gone my way.

I went home so buggered that night and Alison Weeks and Chris Robinson of the taskforce brought in take-away food and we had a superb evening.

Just as the secretariat guided the Wran Committee into a structured approach to resolving key issues, so also it did when it came to

assessing options. In early February 1988, as reflected in the subsequent Wran Report, the committee considered variants of:

- conventional fees schemes (with or without exemptions)
- fees and loan schemes (with government or commercial loan
  arrangements)
- fees with income-contingent loan repayment schemes
- income/asset-contingent fees schemes (exempting those on lower
  incomes).

Each of these options was examined in terms of the following criteria:

- efficiency—impact on overall demand
- administrative simplicity and cost
- equity—impact on socioeconomic composition, access, and capacity of students of different means to be able to pay the charges
- estimates of the revenue implications—short and longer term.

Twelve options resulted and were then ranked in order by each
criterion. For example, in terms of greatest adverse effect on student
demand, fees, even with exemptions, ranked lowest and fees with
government-financed, income-contingent loan repayments ranked best;
but this order was reversed when examining administrative considerations. Detailed analysis by option and criteria led to a summary ranking
table with a 'crude unweighted total' favouring the income-contingent
fees with loan repayment schemes but with income/asset-contingent fees
for the top 20 per cent also coming in near the top of the ranking.

The greatest disadvantage of the option that was to become
HECS was the low level of revenue raised in the first five years.
This concern led the committee to consider, later on, additional
options to meet initial revenue shortfalls. The committee was divided
on which approach to recommend and hence put two options
forward in its report for government consideration:

- a discount to encourage voluntary upfront contributions; or
- compulsory 'upfront' contributions from the top 10 or 20 per
  cent of students on an income and assets test basis. (Committee
  on Higher Education Funding 1988a: 80)

The Wran Committee was keen throughout to combine its student
charges regime with other measures to encourage access, since the
charging system would not do that. So it considered a range of options
including enhancements to AUSTUDY and hypothecating revenue
gained from tuition charges for educational expenditures, including
increased places.

On the basis of the above, the Wran Report contained two main
parts: the first laid out the options for expanding sources of funding

for higher education, and the second outlined 'an integrated reform package'. The discussion in the report included 'vouchers' but rejected them, and in fact the committee had done so very early on, for the obvious reason that a voucher scheme would be inconsistent with the key objectives of growth in number of places and with equity.

Achievement of the various equity and revenue objectives set for HECS would depend crucially on the operational details, that is, the level of the fees set for students and the terms under which those fees would later be repaid through the tax system. Thus the next main part of the Wran Report elaborated on these details. It recommended, on 'historical and overseas' precedents, that the fees for students should be around 20 per cent of the average total costs incurred per student by the Federal Government.

Payment of the greater part of the fees by the government reflected the widely held view that there were substantial benefits to society from higher education, although it was acknowledged that it was virtually impossible to apportion the benefits between those accruing to society and those accruing privately to the individuals who had such an education. The figure of 20 per cent was suggested because it could be related to the level of student fees charged before they were abolished in 1974, and was approximately in line with fees charged by publicly funded universities overseas. This meant that fees per student in 1988 would range from $1200 to $5000 a year, depending on the course studied, and on this basis the committee nominated three fee levels: $3000 a year for full-time students in medicine, dentistry and a few other high-cost courses; $2500 a year for full-time students in engineering, science and several other of the more costly courses; and $1500 for all other students.

The Wran Report recommended that graduates should begin to repay the accumulated debt of their student fees when their annual incomes reached the level of the average annual earnings of all employees in the community (then about $21 500), and that they should then repay the debt through a levy of 2 per cent of their annual taxable income.

The Wran Report estimated that the net gain to revenue from its recommendations would be $445 million in 2001, which would be equivalent to about 50 per cent of the funding gap projected by then in the Green Paper. While the scheme recommended by the Wran Report would have contributed $625 million to revenue by 2001, this would have been offset by the costs of other recommendations in the report—notably an 'access improvement package', involving increased living allowances for students through AUS-TUDY, and abolition of the HEAC that had been introduced only the previous year, in 1987.

The Wran Report also considered how contributions to higher education might be raised from industry, as it is one of the direct beneficiaries of skills developed through higher education. The committee found this issue hard and not central to its concerns; its main recommendation here, however, was for establishment of a 'tripartite body . . . to develop education and training levy arrangements in industry' (p. 76). Behind the scenes, the Department of Prime Minister and Cabinet worked to get the issue referred to another body.

'Some form of employer contribution was an important issue for me. I raised it every meeting, but could never get it up. We didn't know how to do it. So, the philosophy and principle never went anywhere.' (Mike Gallagher)

CONSULTATION

'We called for submissions once. But really, we were a bit of a backroom committee.' (Bob Gregory)

Formal and public consultations were held on the Green Paper. The main aim of the formal consultation, in Dawkins' eyes, was to gain support for his vision of reform in higher education.

Over 600 submissions were received, from higher education institutions, individual academics, business and employer groups, trade unions, community groups and other interested people. DEET's 1987/88 annual report referred to 'wide community discussion' of this report and noted that the 'strong community response . . . lent support to the Government's view that changes to the higher education system were timely and important'. It was noted that there was 'much support for the main points of the proposals, particularly the need for growth and the importance of extending the chance of higher education to those groups that have traditionally been excluded' (1998: 93).

The consultation on the Wran Report was more intense and focused than for the Green Paper, because it was the Wran Report that had grasped the nettle on student charges. The university sector had been critical of the shake-up proposed in the Green Paper. Dawkins had anticipated the controversy that his reforms generally would arouse; so, usually with Paul Hickey of DEET and his senior staff, he consulted informally with a small group of 'reform-minded' university vice-chancellors, dubbed the 'purple circle', and these consultations continued during the deliberations of the Wran Committee. This form of consultation ensured that the higher education sector was aware of the totality of changes being considered, thus adding to the likelihood of acceptance of HECS by the sector.

> *8 May 1988* Went on a bit of a high this week because the Wran Committee report was released. Press conference on Thursday and heaps of publicity . . . On Wednesday lunched with Bruce Chapman to go over arguments and then was briefed in case Wran could not come (because Jill had had their baby) . . . Dawkins was excellent. The wonderful secretariat had prepared a brief for Cabinet which they presented (Alison and Bruce) to it on Tuesday. At a meeting with Howe, he (unlike his staff) said how enthusiastic he was about the report!

> *15 May 1988* Tuesday—my birthday—was hard: division heads meeting followed by child care meeting. In the middle of that the Minister rang wanting a brief on Wran Committee stuff by 5 p.m. Sped off to and from doctor at Civic writing the brief on the bus because I had meetings for the rest of the afternoon.

The summary of public responses to the Wran Committee's proposals released in May 1988 referred to polls showing that two in every three Australians considered that 'students, as major beneficiaries of higher education, should pay at least part of the cost of their courses' (1998c: 2). Suggested alternatives to the committee's proposals mostly provided for others to pay more towards higher education, including the government (i.e. taxpayers generally), industry, or high-income earners in general. A concluding section of the summary, titled 'Refinements to the core proposal', discussed some issues of detail that would figure prominently in later reviews of HECS. These included the costs nominated for different university courses, the threshold level of income or other conditions determining when graduates would start to repay their HECS debts, and the rates at which those repayments should be made, in the form of a percentage surcharge on income tax.

On the release of the Wran Report, negative comments came from students, as expected:

> The NUS Education Vice-President, Ms Kiri Evans, said reports that the Wran Committee on higher education had recommended the introduction of a graduate tax were shocking. 'Even more shocking are reports that Cabinet looked favourably on the Wran recommendations—it will mean the end of universal free tertiary education in Australia, and could well seal the fate of this government', Ms Evans said. (National Union of Students, media statement, 4 May 1988)

The unions were also resistant, wanting more action on levying industry (*ANU Reporter* 13 May 1988), although Dawkins had made sure a big union figure, Laurie Carmichael, understood the issues and would be an advocate for the reforms. The Vice-Chancellors' Committee was positive but cautious, seeing the Wran Report as 'probably the best we can hope for'. Its main concern was that there be no reduction in public funding of universities.

> *'The biggest challenge was to get universities on side, especially after the Green Paper. There was no trust in government.'*
> *(Alison Weeks)*

With the release of the Wran Report, the political consultation began in earnest, particularly to persuade Dawkins' own party to abandon its deep commitment to free university education. This consultation was focused on, though by no means confined to, the biennial National Conference of the ALP scheduled for June 1988. If Dawkins' reforms were to proceed, it was necessary at this conference to have the ALP platform's commitment to a free university education amended.

> *'For Dawkins it was the internal party politics that mattered. If he could sell it to them, then the policy would get through all right.' (Alison Weeks)*

The nature of the public consultation on the Wran Report was conveyed in a paper prepared mainly for delegates to the ALP National Conference. This contained a letter from Wran to conference delegates, arguing the case for the recommendations in his committee's report, and a summary of public responses to that report. His letter emphasised the equity arguments for the committee's recommendations—not surprisingly, in view of his audience. At the heart of these was the fact that a university education was still the privilege of a few, paid for by the community as a whole:

> Not only are higher education students drawn disproportionately from privileged backgrounds, but they themselves tend to be among the more privileged and affluent members of society on graduation . . . a small and relatively privileged section of the community obtains most of the benefits from higher education while the bulk of the costs fall on middle to lower income earners and PAYE taxpayers, most of whom have never attended a higher education institution. (Committee on Higher Education Funding 1988b: 2)

Implicit in these remarks was the evident failure of a system of free university education to widen access to such education, and the case for students themselves to pay more towards their higher education.

Dawkins succeeded in getting revisions to the ALP platform that were sympathetic to his views agreed at the ALP National Conference. Specifically, the new platform no longer contained the commitment to 'free tertiary education' that had been in previous ones, and it contained the following resolution under the heading 'Higher and further education':

> While any kind of compulsory up front fees is rejected, consideration needs to be given to various proposals to provide additional funding including income tax levies on all high income earners, the proposals from the Wran Committee and any other proposals that meet the above principles. (ALP 1988: 74)

MOVING TOWARDS DECISIONS

> The ACCESS [Australian Contribution to the Cost of Education for Students Scheme] higher education funding scheme is the fairest and most innovative education reform package put before the Federal Government in 30 years, Mr Neville Wran, AC, QC, Chairman of the Committee on Higher Education, said today. (Media Release, 5 May 1988)

The Wran Committee recommended what it called an integrated package of measures:

- the 'core proposal' of a higher education contribution scheme with students contributing around 20 per cent of the costs of their courses over time, subject to capacity to pay
- a set of financial initiatives to expand participation of the disadvantaged through improvements to AUSTUDY and other student assistance schemes
- establishment of a tripartite body to develop appropriate arrangements for industry contributions to education and training
- abolition of the Higher Education Administrative Charge.

Important too was the recommendation that the proceeds of the higher education contribution scheme be placed in a dedicated trust fund to be spent only on increasing the number of student places and improving student assistance under AUSTUDY.

Dawkins issued a press release: 'Its own basic solution is without precedent in the world. This is largely because the Committee adhered strictly to the injunction in its terms of reference to have regard to the social as well as educational implications of its recommendations' (Dawkins 1988b: 5).

Dawkins played the politics hard, from the Wran announcements through the ALP Platform Committee on education, to the ALP National Conference in June and in the lead-up to the August budget. Fear of Gough Whitlam's negativism about any charges led

Walsh eyes uni fees to keep the deficit down

Hawke hints ... reverse ter...

Ministers differ on tertiary fees

range of small proposal to reintroduce fees for university and college have surfaced yet, but he would be aiming for something in the hundreds of millions of dollars range. Senator Walsh's depart-

...ates of ...t the tri- ...ave to be ...illion and ...determined

Opposition college ...gath... ...student fees: Ryan

...quire it to monitor the effect of the charge on different categories of students, and consider research commissioned by the Commonwealth Tertiary Education Commission. The committee is chaired by the CTEC chairman, Mr Hugh Hudson, and includes MPs and representatives of the Federal Education Department, the universities and students.

University R...

...posal ...ding ...defeat

...ced ...es

Borrowing the cost of higher education

...TRALIAN
Budget deficit.
...ts EPAC

IT was for Finance's proposal ...ure tuition fees in universities

Academics warn Govt on lack of tertiary funds

It is neither surprising nor deplorable that these considerations should influence the thinking of Labor politicians. However, as other members of the Labor Party have ...ted out, the issue is not entirely

Haw... Caucu... move ...against fees ...ision

...e upsets L

Walsh pushes ...an scheme for

Hawke backs away from move to bring back tertiary fees

Tertiary-education fees as a ...to save public money

Walsh to give Caucus ...

...lash with ...
is ...
...ttle to mak...

would hurt

...body urges
Graduate tax ...hange
tertiary fee...
are possible

education

Green Paper on higher education ref...

...ation of m...

Graduate ...
win for Dawk...

L – Dawkins
...wkins starts
graduate tax
hard sell to ALP
Tertiary

...deregu...ation of...

Dawk...
shake up univer...

Budget 88
Education

when a s... reaches $22 Progres... arrange... through

...wkins ...ts fee... ...ssue ba... ...en agen...
...1983–2

...ducation
...ibs
Debates across th...

...opp...ose

The Opposition will not oppose the ...ederal Government's controversial tax Ral... ...sation would jo...

Ryan puts strong case to ...ation against tertiary fees ...ary tax: ...ucus would jo... ...ppositio... ...gives

Labor's ...
...p: the political ...ertiary-ta...
...r tertiary fees ...ate tax pro...

The press

Political journalists with the main Australian newspapers were also important players in the HECS debate, in that they drew attention to political sensitivities surrounding tertiary fees. For example, the controversial proposal of Senator Walsh in 1985 to re-introduce some form of charge for tertiary students, and the differences of view on this within the Cabinet and ALP, received a lot of attention from leading political journalists in February and March that year.

Press headlines provide insights into the nature of the political debate, and indirectly convey in retrospect the extent of the challenge faced by Dawkins when he introduced HECS: 'Hawke hints Caucus might reverse tertiary fee decision' (Louise Dodson, *Australian Financial Review*, 17 May 1985: 5); 'Hawke upsets Left on tertiary fees' (Howard Conkey, *Canberra Times*, 17 May 1985: 1); 'Hawke facing caucus move against fees' (Ian Davis, *Age*, 20 May 1985: 5); and finally, 'Hawke backs away from move to bring back tertiary fees' (Amanda Buckley and Mike Steketee, *Sydney Morning Herald*, 21 May 1985: 1). It was thus not surprising that when Dawkins introduced his HECS proposals in 1988, the press continued to focus on the politics of the issues, though in the context of Dawkins' broader proposals for change in the tertiary sector: 'Dawkins starts graduate tax hard sell to ALP' (Donald Greenlees, *Australian*, 22 August 1988: 3); 'Graduate tax big win for Dawkins' (Robert Reid, *Australian*, 24 August 1988: 6); and 'Labor's tertiary-tax plan "very brave"' (Penelope Layland, *Canberra Times*, 6 September 1988: 2).

In the lead-up to the publication of the Wran Report, the press reaction had been largely favourable, with positive comments from key commentators. Once the report was released, newspapers gave it much publicity; they publicised the negative reactions from many stakeholder groups, but also gave much space to supportive pieces in editorials and commentaries.

For example, under the headline 'Wran Graduate Tax Plan Staunchly Opposed', the *Australian Financial Review* said: 'The Wran Committee's proposal to raise $635 million a year by the end of the century by requiring tertiary students to pay a 2 per cent graduate tax has hit an immediate wall of opposition from students, the ALP Caucus, the business community and the trade union movement' (Wayne Burns, *AFR* 6 May 1988: 6).

The *Australian*, on the same day on its front page, while

noting opposition to the scheme, had political comment from Paul Kelly which was strongly in favour of the proposals: 'The Labor Party has bitten on the user-pays principle in tertiary education. It has broken through the futile political debate about fees with a new concept that should win party approval and transform higher education funding' (*Australian*, 6 May 1988: 1). Kelly concluded his article this way:

> It is merely another test of Labor's judgment and nerve. At a time when the party has jelly legs about firm decisions— asset sales, spending cuts, waterfront reforms—a bit of sensible leadership has been brought to bear in the tertiary funding area. If the party cannot wear this then it had been [*sic*] better sign out in the Parliament House visitor's book next Monday.

Dawkins to gain a commitment, if a shaky one, that Whitlam would not pour cold water on the proposal, at least not publicly.

29 July 1988 All we have been working for since last November has come to fruition in the Budget process. *All* of the Minister's [Howe's] packages have gone on to success. A fantastic record of achievement plus Dawkins' Graduate Tax. Week before this one spent half the week waiting for Cabinet, ERC or Social and Family Policy Committee to call.

The main substantive difference between the scheme the government actually adopted in the budget of August 1988 and the Wran recommendations was to not vary the charge according to course cost. (This decision was later turned back nearer to the Wran recommendation.) This was a reaction to Caucus concerns, in particular about poorer students who were likely to be risk-averse and so discouraged from taking more expensive courses (e.g. medicine and engineering compared with arts and law), and there is some evidence that the department put this case on equity grounds.

The government exempted students enrolled in basic nurse education courses (until 1993), adult education and continuing education students, and students enrolled in non-award courses; it also exempted 15 000 postgraduate scholarships, including those for the professional development of teachers. It opted for the discount of 15 per cent for students who paid their fees upfront.

To keep universities on side, $10m was allocated each year to help higher education institutions meet their administrative costs in implementing the scheme.

4 June 1988 At airport went straight to Golden Wing lounge to start preparations for talk I had to give with others that night to 500 students on Wran Committee proposals. Met Bruce there. Both in an agitated state so spent the hour or so on the direct flight to Adelaide preparing our talks . . . Also speaking was Ken Davidson (journalist), Kiri Evans (the formidable student representative) and Hugh Stretton. Bruce, Frank Milne (ANU) and I were on the other side. Debate went on for three hours or so, each of us speaking for ten minutes and then questions from the 500-odd attendees. I answered a lot of the questions. Poor Bruce, being the male economist quoting facts all the time, didn't come through so well . . . 8.30 a.m. next morning, on talkback radio for half an hour with Kiri Evans . . .

This initiative was huge at a time when the government was still concerned with the budget deficit. It amounted to an increase of almost $1 billion being committed to higher education over three years, on the basis of an expected stream of HECS revenue into the future. The number of higher education places was forecast to increase by 50 per cent in the first five years.

IMPLEMENTATION

'Dealings with the Tax Office appeared to me to be a classic example of obfuscation, obstruction and hindrance in bureaucratic politics, but for quite good reasons that I understood later.'
(Bruce Chapman)

As HECS involves payments by students that relate to the level of their incomes, it seemed obvious to those who were developing HECS that a simple and efficient method for collecting such payments would be through the tax system. The ATO was initially opposed to doing this, however, and the account of how it changed its mind illustrates some important and not uncommon issues in policy implementation.

The first discussions with the ATO occurred as part of the process of interdepartmental consultation that normally precedes submission of a proposal to Cabinet. Although implementation of a policy is commonly seen as an 'administrative' issue to be settled among officials within the bureaucracy, on this occasion responsibility for the initial discussions with the Tax Office, curiously, was given to Bruce Chapman, who commented that at the time he had 'not

much experience of how this should be done . . . [and] no understanding of the policy process' (Chapman 1996a: 13).

> 'It was a salutary experience, one of those things in your career
> that turns out to be a turning point in an understanding of how
> things work. I now laugh at my image: a wet-behind-the ears aca-
> demic strolling cheerfully to the ATO with the unquestioned
> conviction that if a policy was good, bureaucrats would naturally
> jump at the chance of implementing it. I projected that they'd
> leap up and down with enthusiasm and say, "what a terrific
> idea, Bruce, we'd just love to be involved!" I was much younger
> then.
>   'My recollection of this first meeting is as follows. I argued
> that a charge for higher education was justified. I explained the
> merits of collecting such a charge depending on graduates' future
> incomes, and pushed that for these things to happen the ATO
> was the natural (the only) collection institution available. The
> ATO, I think I said, had the unique advantages of knowing
> what graduates' incomes were and being able to easily make the
> relevant deductions from salaries. I probably said something like:
> "This is a great opportunity for path-breaking policy reform".
>   'At the end of my short presentation I can remember thinking
> there would be no doubt they would be keen to be involved in the
> development of the policy. I did what most of us frequently do: I
> projected that they would agree to what I thought was the ob-
> vious (i.e. what I wanted). However, it soon became clear that
> this was not the case. The more senior of the two (I could tell,
> because his seat was higher) said: "The Tax Office collects taxes,
> not debts. This is a basic principle." Their raising the issue of
> "principle" seemed to be the end of the conversation, because a
> "principle"—by definition—is something that can never be compro-
> mised. I left the ATO disheartened, with my confused tail
> between my legs, and my racket in tatters. But I knew I had to
> come back, maybe many times.
>   'Preparing for the next meeting I decided to ignore the diffi-
> cult issue of what a principle actually means, and instead
> planned on asking them to outline the practical implementation
> issues. At this second meeting they came up with many problems,
> such as: "People avoid taxes. What does this scheme do about
> that?"; or "People die. How can we collect their debt if this hap-
> pens? We don't have death duties in this country."
>   'I hadn't thought much about these issues at the time. At
> the meeting I was not able to respond convincingly and felt even
> more disheartened and frustrated. I thought about these questions

and decided to address them at the third meeting. I wanted to address the empirical significance of adverse possibilities, and what their existence might mean for the viability of the policy. It seemed to me that none of the practical difficulties raised by the ATO were important. They probably knew I was right and, as a consequence, reverted back to the principle: "The Tax Office does not collect debt". Then a critical thing happened.

'In a coffee break from the discussion ("battle" is probably the right word), the senior man asked me, by way of friendly conversation, who was on the Wran Committee. I said Bob Gregory (who they seemed to approve of), Mike Gallagher (no opinion was expressed), and Meredith Edwards. The mention of the last changed everything.

'The senior official's demeanour changed radically, and much to the negative, at the mention of Meredith's name. He turned to his offsider and said "We're stuffed". They seemed then to wave a white flag; the Wran Committee had won the Wimbledon final, after being two sets to nil down.

'Later I came to appreciate why Meredith Edwards being on the Wran Committee was critical to the ATO's assent. It was because, unknown to me, Meredith Edwards had been fundamentally involved in the institution of the non-custodial parenting support scheme. ATO was already involved in doing things that were not just about taxes, and could be described as "debt collection". In other words, the "principle" of the ATO not being a debt collector had already been significantly compromised well before I turned up arguing for HECS.

'Essentially this was the end of my involvement with the ATO with respect of HECS. ATO officials came to the Wran Committee for discussion about administrative arrangements, but there was not strong opposition. The administrative issue was resolved.' (Bruce Chapman)

The ATO offered two reasons why it should not be responsible for implementing HECS: such a task would conflict with its traditional functions, and in particular with the principle that it should not be a debt collection agency; and, perhaps somewhat inconsistently with this argument, some of the possible debts that could arise under HECS would be difficult to collect. These would include debts of students emigrating or dying after graduation, and debts of those graduates who evaded their obligations in the same way as some other taxpayers evade their tax obligations.

These arguments were successfully countered, essentially because of a precedent for debt collection by the ATO, and doubts about the significance of any bad debts. Not long before the HECS issue arose, the ATO had become involved in collecting payments from non-custodial parents for child maintenance (see Chapter 3). The way in which this fact entered the argument about the Tax Office's principled opposition to involvement with HECS as described above

Further, there was little evidence to indicate that the possible losses through bad debts from defaulting or dying graduates would be significant when compared with the gains to revenue from HECS and the obvious efficiencies from collecting HECS payments through the tax system.

The ATO's initially reluctant acquiescence in implementing HECS turned within a few years into enthusiastic support for such an arrangement, due in no small measure to Paul Keating's support. When in 1992 it was proposed that the ATO should collect certain other debts from students, related to student income support, its response was 'completely different'. The official discussions with the ATO to arrange collection of these debts, based on the system operating by then for HECS, revealed that it had become an enthusiastic supporter of the HECS arrangement: 'in contradistinction to the 1988 discussion, a range of HECS promotional material (such as pens, balloons, a video and a board game) were offered as evidence for the ATO's commitment to the [HECS] scheme' (Chapman 1996a: 14–15).

> 'Some time later [after HECS] I had to confront the ATO with a policy development similar to HECS. In 1992 I recommended that the Government introduce the Austudy Loan Supplement. This also required the ATO to collect debt. This time when I went to the ATO to discuss the proposal the action stung me: "Not a problem" one of the same officials said and I nearly fell off the chair. He then said: "Do you have a HECS pen?". He offered me an ATO biro-type implement which had written on it: "HECS—the ATO Working for You". He was clearly pleased that there was such a thing. He followed this up with: "Have you seen our HECS video?". And he went on to say proudly that this was shown in most Australian high schools to Year 12 students so they knew what would happen to them with respect to university charges and how they would be paid. This was followed with some HECS balloons and a HECS board game. I left the ATO in a daze, struggling to hold my video, pens, balloons and board games.
>
> 'On reflection it was not hard to understand why the ATO was now embracing HECS and the Austudy Loans Supplement. A government department is right to resist new administrative

arrangements, particularly if it is obvious that they will involve greater staff input, as HECS did. After all, they may not get the required additional staff and this would mean harder work for those there . . . If a public servant's role is partly about avoiding screw-ups it makes sense not to get involved too unquestioningly, and this they certainly weren't.

'I consider that the ATO acted perfectly reasonably, indeed rationally, both in the barriers they erected, and their eventual acceptance and ownership of HECS. This institution showed itself to be a model of cautious and progressive administration, and we should acknowledge gratefully their professionalism.'
(Bruce Chapman)

There were many strands to implementation. One was continuing to confront hostile universities where Paul Hickey from DEET played a key role. Dawkins had to go back to Cabinet to gain additional dollars for implementation to placate the university sector. Consultation and 'selling' took place beyond the budget announcements as implementation progressed beyond the university sector, especially within the ALP, and to student groups as well as to ACOSS, the Australian Council of Trade Unions (ACTU), the Business Council and union groups. Dawkins wrote to every enrolled student on why the scheme was necessary and how it would work.

Alongside the above, constitutional issues were requiring the close attention of legal advisers. The Minister, if not the government, could see good political reasons not to have HECS regarded as a tax, even though that would have given the Commonwealth the needed consitutional authority for HECS. Dennis Rose, Solicitor-General in the Attorney-General's Department, was brought in for advice. When Rose suggested that the part of the Constitution dealing with 'benefits for students' should be used, Dawkins and his advisers laughed. Dawkins, however, did not laugh once Rose explained how this could be done.

'The Commonwealth could provide grants to the states for universities subject to the states requiring universities to charge fees upfront. The Commonwealth would then provide the (deferred) loan to students, repayable when income exceeds the stated sum.'
(Dennis Rose)

This example (as with child support), illustrates how legal advice can impact on actual decisions, especially to get around constitutional difficulties, and can lead to a change to the conceptual base of a scheme to make it workable and/or politically acceptable. Rose saw his job as working out how to do 'indirectly' what was wanted, if that could not be done directly.

Students did start a High Court challenge to the legislation, but backed off when they realised that if they won on constitutional grounds, the Commonwealth would turn to its tax power.

> *'The disconnection of policy advice from the department in charge of implementation made putting the systems in place that much harder.' (Mike Gallagher)*

Given the short time from the Cabinet decision on HECS to the start of the scheme—less than five months—and some resistance from those implementing because they were not involved in the policy development process, the process was helped considerably by the continuity of a few key players, such as Chris Robinson, who had been a member of the Wran Committee secretariat and went on to head the HECS implementation unit in the department, and Paul Hickey, as well as a dedicated implementation taskforce under the experienced leadership of Peter Grant.

This experience with HECS illustrates two important points about the realities of policy implementation. First, officials asked to implement new policies will often be inclined to be cautious initially and to see 'difficulties' for reasons that may be quite rational from individual or organisational perspectives: apart from uncertainties about whether acquiring new responsibilities will make life more difficult, there may also be uncertainties, in an environment of tight budgets and scarce resources, about whether the additional resources needed to perform new tasks properly will be provided. Second, the course of the argument about implementation of HECS illustrates the significance that established practice and precedent can acquire in the bureaucracy. The ATO was initially reluctant to administer HECS because this conflicted with an established concept of the ATO's role. A precedent for extending that role (its recent involvement in the administration of child support) became a telling reason for also taking on HECS, and once this had been done, the ATO's role in HECS became a good reason why it should also take on similar responsibilities a little later with debts relating to student income support.

EVALUATION

Several evaluations have been done of HECS, beginning with one undertaken in 1989, soon after the scheme was introduced (Robertson et al. 1990). This study was funded and guided by the government through DEET. Its general aim was 'to seek to understand the motivation of those deciding not to participate or continue in higher education, including the impact of the HECS on their decision' (letter, Milligan to Chapman, 4 May 1989). It was thus addressing the central issue of HECS, access to higher education, and in particular a widespread apprehension at the time HECS was introduced that the charges it imposed on students would deter some from starting or continuing with higher education.

The study was undertaken by academics from Flinders and Curtin Universities and it examined effects of HECS on the participation of students in higher education in Victoria and Western Australia, and in particular on the extent to which the types of charges introduced by HECS deterred such participation. It was based on a questionnaire survey, and it concluded that HECS had little effect on 1989 undergraduate enrolments: only 2 per cent of potential entrants to the institutions surveyed cited HECS as important in a decision not to enrol, and only 5 per cent of undergraduates cited it important in a decision not to re-enrol; about 10 per cent of potential postgraduates cited HECS as an important reason for not re-enrolling. Mature-age students and those whose parents had lower educational qualifications were more prominent among the relatively small numbers of students deterred by HECS charges. The quantitative impact 'was largely confined to the post-graduate area, and even here, the proportion deterred by HECS was less than 10 per cent' (Robertson et al. 1990: ii).

A few years later, in 1992, the Higher Education Council initiated a study of the effects of HECS on the higher education aspirations of Year 12 students and adults 'perceived as potentially disadvantaged' (NBEET 1992). The council was a high-level body established to advise the Minister on educational issues, and it was required to report annually on the operation of HECS. In response to concerns expressed by the National Board of Employment, Education and Training about effects of HECS on the particular groups mentioned, it commissioned a firm of consultants (Ernst & Young) to survey students in New South Wales, Victoria, Queensland and Western Australia. Ernst & Young were assisted in the work by academics from the Higher Education Advisory and Research Unit at Monash University. The terms of reference for the study sought to build on previous studies of the impact of HECS and to provide 'a deeper qualitative understanding' of how it affected students' decisions about studying.

The findings of the study were broadly similar to those of Robertson and colleagues (1990)—in other words, that HECS seemed to have only marginal effects on the intentions of those surveyed. It concluded that, for Year 12 students, it was unlikely that there were any groups for which HECS was 'a critically important influence on decisions about participating in higher education; and that for the 'potentially disadvantaged' adults surveyed, HECS was only a 'middle ranking factor' among all those that seemed to influence decisions about higher education study (p. xii).

The findings of these two studies, that the introduction of student charges for higher education had not significantly changed access to such education, were broadly consistent with data on trends in the composition of the higher education student body collected by the Australian Council of Educational Research. These data showed that the socioeconomic composition of 18-year-old students, for example, was about the same in 1988, before HECS was introduced, as it was five years later in 1993. More specifically, they showed that while enrolments of such students increased over this period, the proportions coming from families of high, medium or low incomes were about the same at the end of the period as at the beginning (Chapman and Smith 1994: 14).

Thus empirical analysis of the effects of HECS seemed to support a conclusion that 'even a radical movement away from a no charge system can be instituted without jeopardising the participation of disadvantaged potential students; this is all traceable to income contingent repayment' (Chapman 1996b: 14).

CONCLUSIONS

The story of HECS illustrates how the 'right' mixture of ideas and expertise can produce a radical and enduring policy change. Unlike many other radical policy changes, it had a relatively brief gestation and a quick birth: less than eighteen months elapsed between the central ideas behind HECS beginning to take shape and the scheme starting operation in January 1989, around ten months up to Cabinet decision. There are several reasons for such an enduring policy emerging so quickly.

- It was driven by an energetic and influential minister, John Dawkins, who became closely involved in the policy process, even though he started off with a relatively open mind on the specific charging regime.
- The analytical stage of the process had much intellectual depth and substance, both through the involvement of academic economists from the Australian National University—notably Bruce Chapman as consultant to Dawkins (for a crucial period Chap-

man was engaged in the process full-time) and the hard-working and able service of a selected group of public servants.

- Implementation was administratively fairly simple, once the main elements of the policy had been determined (and after some bureaucratic resistance on issues of 'principle' had been overcome).
- Fundamentally, and with the benefit of hindsight, HECS was in many respects an 'idea whose time has come' (see Kingdon 1995: 1ff.): it was recognised as a pragmatic response to a situation in which demand for university places was increasing, government funding of universities was contracting, and some form of student contribution towards university costs began to seem both equitable and efficient.

The contrast between the attempts of Walsh and Dawkins to put university fees in some form on the agenda is worth examining. The story of HECS and its policy development is a story about the role of a strong minister who read the environment well. Unlike Walsh, who explicitly advocated the introduction of fees, which would have led to increased government revenue, Dawkins put a different slant on the problem. He did highlight the need for increased revenue to be raised from within the sector, but alongside the need for an increase in places. In addition, he did not propose a specific solution initially. Instead, he established the Wran Committee in December 1997 to consider this question in greater depth, after placing the funding issues in a broader economic and social context.

In one sense, the issue of charging for university education is ever present and timeless. It is part of the broader issue of university funding, and thus is as old as universities themselves. The personalities involved in the development of HECS included not only a reformist minister, who brilliantly played the politics, but also the influential academics and bureaucrats who took part. While many others were also involved, this chapter has shown how these people variously contributed drive, political judgment and public persuasion, ideas and theory, rigorous analysis and an understanding of administrative practicalities in what was, with hindsight, the right mixture to produce a successful and enduring outcome, at the right time. The chapter has thus highlighted that effective policy-making requires an artful mixture of process, people, politics and analysis.

WORKING NATION
CHRONOLOGY OF EVENTS NOVEMBER 1992 TO MAY 1994

1992

November Speech by Bernie Fraser calling for a longer-term policy framework on unemployment.

1993

February Prime Minister Keating's pre-election statement.

March Labor Government re-elected.

May Committee on Employment Opportunities announced.

June Speech by Beazley to National Press Club on need to reduce long-term unemployment.

July Call for submissions by CEO.

August–October Caucus Taskforce consultations with report to CEO in October.

December Green Paper *Restoring Full Employment* released.

1994

January Consultations by CEO on Green Paper.

January–February Interdepartmental working groups design policy options.

February Committee of secretaries formed.

February The first of several meetings of special Ad Hoc Committee of Cabinet ministers chaired by the PM.

March–April Cabinet submission on public consultations and submissions. Drafting of White Paper by Taskforce and staff at PM&C.

May PM tables White Paper, *Working Nation*, in Parliament. Release of report on public consultations and submissions.

Chapter Five

Long-term unemployment policy: From Green Paper to Working Nation

Unemployment is one of the most intractable political, social and economic problems to have faced policy-makers in recent decades, and reducing it is a complex and multifaceted process. As in the other three areas discussed so far, responsibility for formulating and implementing unemployment policy crossed different arenas of government decision-making, requiring agreement and coordination among a disparate collection of official players.

There are also numerous interests outside government with a stake in the unemployment issue and government responses to it. Unions, employers, social welfare groups, the employed, the unemployed and the communities in which they live are all affected. Paid work is the primary means of making personal incomes in Australia and so is a central aspect of people's financial and social lives. When employment opportunities are absent the state and non-profit institutions must incur the burden of supporting those out of work, and unemployed people suffer hardship and loss of self-esteem. The economy also fails to exploit valuable productive resources, so operates less effectively.

As unemployment has risen over the last two decades, so too has expenditure on alleviating the problem and, hence, interest in evaluating the efforts of governments to reduce unemployment.

Much analysis has focused on assessing the effectiveness of labour market programs, the impact of income support policies, and the contribution of wage policies to unemployment. Less interest has been shown in the processes by which these policies are developed and the implications of these for policy effectiveness, efficiency and sustainability.

This chapter examines the processes surrounding the formulation, implementation and evaluation of employment policies starting with the development of the Green Paper *Restoring Full Employment* and culminating in the 1994 White Paper *Working Nation*, the first White Paper on unemployment since *Full Employment and Growth* in 1945. The focus is on the policies introduced to assist the long-term unemployed (LTU)—defined as people unemployed for over one year—to get back into work.

HISTORY AND CONTEXT

Since the 1970s, unemployment rates in most Western economies have 'ratcheted' up during and following each economic downturn. In the early 1990s the rate reached its highest level in Australia since the Great Depression, with over a million people officially measured as out of work; by early 1993 it was 12 per cent. The LTU made up around 45 per cent of those receiving unemployment allowances at this time.

During the 1993 federal election the Opposition made much of the Labor Government's alleged failures of economic management, manifested in the record unemployment rate. In response the government promised to make employment its 'key national priority' if re-elected. Prime Minister Keating's pre-election statement on 10 February 1993 placed this priority in a context: 'Confronting the reality of unemployment means providing a social net to ease the hardship. It also means providing all the training opportunities we can. But above all else it means we must create more growth' (Keating 1993: 8).

It was in this political and economic context that the government announced its intention to develop, through a formal policy process, a comprehensive strategy to address unemployment. The outcome of this process was a discussion paper or Green Paper, issued at the end of 1993, followed the next May by a budget document, the White Paper, presenting the government's policy package.

The White Paper allocated a record amount of over $2 billion in 1995/96 to help the unemployed get jobs—a reform package which, for the first time in Australia, included an effective guarantee of employment for the LTU in the form of the 'Job Compact'. The package included individual case management for the LTU, the contracting out of state-funded labour market assistance (other than through the Commonwealth Employment Service), and substantial changes to the design of the income support system for the unemployed. Unlike the Green Paper that preceded it, this document also addressed regional and industry policies.

Since the present Coalition Government's initiatives on the LTU could be argued to be a development of particular reforms in the *Working Nation* case, such as individualised and contracted case management and performance incentives for private providers (Grant 1998; Stromback and Dockery 1998), an analysis of *Working Nation* is important for understanding the policy ideas, issues and conflicts that underlie the present system of assistance to the unemployed in Australia.

STRUCTURE AND PLAYERS

A theme of this book is that the process by which policy analysis and development is undertaken can be as important as the policy content itself in achieving desired reform.

> *'The feeling outside the government was that this all was very late . . . that the Labor Party, which was traditionally worried about unemployment, was taking a long time getting to this point. Outsiders would have thought that this process would have started much earlier than it did.' (Bob Gregory)*

In May 1993 the Labor Government formed the **Committee on Employment Opportunities** (CEO) to steer the Green Paper process. It also established a supporting **taskforce of officials** from across many Federal Government agencies. The committee consisted of both 'insiders' and 'outsiders': three senior public servants—the Secretary of PM&C, Dr Michael Keating (chair), and the heads of DSS and DEET; three academic experts (economics and social work); and a senior adviser from the PM's office.

It is interesting to consider this composition. Having three powerful insiders—none of them from Treasury—on a high-powered economic committee could reflect the Prime Minister's disenchantment with Treasury's previous performance (see J. Edwards 1996: 384 *et passim*). The three departmental heads had the skills and resources to test the practicality of suggested policies and were chosen to ensure continuity from policy development to implementation. Including academic experts, rather than representatives of the interests of the unemployed, suggests a desire to gain expert advice based on relevant research. There could also have been a desire to avoid unduly contentious perspectives. The fact that the CEO included the Prime Minister's social policy adviser and that its chair was the head of PM&C suggests the PM's keenness to ensure that it did not go off the rails, while giving its members some freedom to play with ideas and policy directions. Unlike other committees set up by ministers, such as the Wran Committee (Chapter 4), the Prime Minister would have found it most difficult, on receiving a final report, not to endorse it.

> *'What is remarkable is that Treasury and Finance were not on it. Interestingly, Treasury took this very much to heart . . . and used it as a bit of soul searching.' (Mary Ann O'Loughlin)*

The composition of the CEO may have appeared to some to be limited in its perspectives, but it did lead to a deep level of debate and a wide search for deliverable options. The supporting taskforce comprised subject-matter experts, with policy and evaluation expertise from line departments, some central agency staff, and an ABS representative, as well as experienced policy leadership. Both structures gained from an existing store of knowledge and breadth of vision. This was very different from the more normal process of a line department undertaking policy development, culminating in a Cabinet submission on behalf of its minister, with or without an IDC process.

External representation on the CEO allowed a wider canvassing of options and the building up of public debate by key individuals who were not constrained by their position in the government service; more radical options could be canvassed than if there had been reliance entirely on an internal process. Broader membership could have engendered a further broadening of view, but the CEO could also have become driven by more sectional interests regarding outcomes, as well as possibly impractical prescriptions.

Perhaps not so evident is the importance of the CEO's composition and that of its supporting taskforce in providing a 'whole-of-government approach' to the issue. This was fairly new at this time and was probably the first time it had occurred across so many departmental interests.

The taskforce also continued into the White Paper phase and had several important functions:

- communicating the objectives of the CEO to the cross-departmental working groups
- continuing to project the evaluation and research evidence into the working group discussions

- maintaining the overall vision and policy links within specialist working groups
- playing honest broker as central agency staff (or secondees)
- improving communication across agencies, as former and returning members of line departments.

In many policy exercises of this kind, continuity is not achieved because the review is external to the bureaucracy while the response and policy construction is internal.

In the production of the White Paper, the taskforce and the Department of Prime Minister and Cabinet in which it was located clearly demonstrated the 'honest broker' role that a central agency can play by bringing together competing cross-portfolio interests, pushing towards common objectives, and producing a draft report for government decision. The White Paper was ultimately a prime ministerial statement, though the contribution of portfolio ministers and their advisers cannot be overestimated. But PM&C's role in drafting it gave it more influence than it would otherwise have had.

Interdepartmental Working Groups were set up in both the Green and White Paper processes. Working within the above organisational structure, they allowed more fully informed discussion of options and provided an important measure of coherence, which is essential for policy development that crosses departmental boundaries.

To a large degree in the Green Paper working groups, the usual policy development roles of line departments and central agencies were reversed; in this process, the taskforce and PM&C staff were more often the purveyors of the key Green Paper directions, which were then tested for their practicality by line departments during the following White Paper process. This reflected the need for an interdepartmental approach to the problem, but the taskforce itself included departmental representatives, from Treasury and elsewhere.

The White Paper Working Groups worked for an overarching **Committee of Secretaries**. By early 1994 secretaries not represented on the CEO were agitating for more formal input. The head of PM&C therefore formed a Committee of Secretaries to coordinate policy and settle disputes on technical issues before ministerial consideration. The three secretaries on this committee carried their involvement into this forum and were joined by three other secretaries from Finance, Treasury, and Industry, Science and Technology, who were eager to become involved. This committee did not meet often, nor did it need to, but it played a useful role in resolving a number of disputes, in particular about the costing of policy proposals. It also ensured that the policy rationale and directions of the Green Paper were carried to the highest level in the central agencies charged with fiscal policy, and ensured the consistency and coordination of policy across portfolios.

Once key memoranda had been written and approved by the Committee of Secretaries, they went before a ministerial committee which narrowed down the options. This left line departments, under ministerial guidance, to take over the implementation phase.

A committee of ministers, the **Ad Hoc Committee of Cabinet**, was formed in February 1994 to decide policy for the White Paper. Ministers in this committee had a high degree of common purpose, reflecting the period of community debate and the publication of the Green Paper. Their level of informed debate was also enhanced by the fact that the committee contained four previous or current employment ministers.

The Ad Hoc Committee's membership heavily overlapped that of the **Expenditure Review Committee of Cabinet** (the key Cabinet committee responsible for deciding annually where budget cuts would come from) and now, with Kim Beazley as Finance Minister, was crucial to the prospects for cross-portfolio policy design. Only ministers close to the centre have the overview and power to make decisions that span the range of government activity; the prime ministerial role is to finally resolve entrenched disagreement and move from policy discussion to policy decision. The Ad Hoc Committee agreed on the broad outlines of policy reform and determined the broad aggregate dollar outlay involved.

It is worth noting that alongside this bureaucratic and political structure there existed a specially established **Caucus Employment Taskforce**, co-chaired by backbenchers Wayne Swan and Rod Sawford. This taskforce facilitated the work of the expert CEO by undertaking consultations and making available to the CEO an early copy of their report as the basis for an exchange of views.

THE PLAYERS

Politicians

Baldwin, Peter	Minister for Social Security
Beazley, Kim	Minister for Employment, Education and Training 1993
	Minister for Finance 1993–96
Crean, Simon	Minister for Employment, Education and Training 1993–96
Keating, Paul	Prime Minister
Sawford, Rod	Co-Chair, Caucus Employment Taskforce

Swan, Wayne	Co-Chair, Caucus Employment Taskforce

Public servants

Blunn, Tony	Secretary, DSS and Member of CEO
Briggs, Lynelle	Head, Social Policy Division, DSS
Campbell, Ian	Division Head, DEET
Edwards, Dr Meredith	Head of Taskforce on Employment Opportunities, Deputy Secretary, Department of PM&C
Grant, Peter	Deputy Secretary, DEET
Hickey, Paul	Head, Higher Education Division, DEET
Keating, Dr Michael	Secretary, PM&C; Chair, CEO
Lindenmayer, Ian	Deputy Secretary, DEET
Moore, Stephen	Senior officer, DEET
Pech, Jocelyn	Senior officer, DSS
Ryan, Dr Chris	Branch head, DEET
Stuart, Andrew	Member of Taskforce on Employment Opportunities as a senior official from DEET
Volker, Derek	Secretary, DEET 1993; member, CEO
Wilson, Serena	Senior officer, DSS

Ministerial advisers

Chapman, Dr Bruce	Consultant to DEET and Prime Minister's Office, September 1994
O'Loughlin, Mary Ann	Senior adviser, Social Policy, to the Prime Minister
Phillips, David	Senior adviser, Minister for Employment, Education and Training, 1991–93

Academics

Carter, Prof. Jan	Member, CEO
Gregory, Prof. Bob	Member, CEO
Hughes, Prof. Barry	Member, CEO

Other

Fraser, Bernie	Governor of Reserve Bank

IDENTIFYING THE ISSUES

In the early 1990s, when existing policy on unemployment was widely perceived as inadequate, the government made several policy announcements in its budgets and in economic statements in an attempt to alleviate the problem. Typically this led to increases in spending on those labour market programs that monitoring information suggested had the better outcomes for the client—all part of an incremental approach to assisting the unemployed. There was no obvious solution to what seemed an intractable problem.

One influential event in the period leading up to the 1993 election was a speech given by the Governor of the Reserve Bank, Bernie Fraser, in November 1992. Fraser called for a longer-term policy framework to be developed involving people outside government but with the government in the driving seat: 'Perhaps it is time, being almost 50 years since the White Paper on "Full Employment in Australia" appeared, that we need a similar paper on growth and related issues' (Fraser 1992: 264). This suggestion was taken up as one of several options in a brief from the head of PM&C, Dr Michael Keating, which was presented to the Prime Minister the day after the election. Fraser's public remarks were significant because from that point it was difficult for the Prime Minister to address the problem internally, which could well have been his instinct—now there was pressure on him to involve players outside the government.

Unemployment ran counter to the social values of the ALP, so it was no surprise that on re-election the Labor Government gave a strong commitment to deal with the unemployment issue. But there were also political reasons for putting radical employment reforms on the agenda.

THE NATURE OF THE PROBLEM

It is hard to disentangle all the factors that led to the problem of long-term (as distinct from high) unemployment being placed firmly on the agenda. But several forces were operating to ensure that politicians could not ignore the problem.

A crucial contribution was the identification by a few academic labour market researchers of the urgency of reducing long-term unemployment. The work of Dr Bruce Chapman and his associates at the ANU formed the basis for much of the underlying economic rationale for policy action. Chapman and his colleagues (1992, 1993), projecting LTU rates for the 1990s, pointed out that even with highly optimistic economic growth forecasts, the numbers of individuals in LTU would not decline significantly from high post-recession levels. Economic growth alone was not enough to solve the problem.

Immediately after the election in March 1993, Chapman and policy advisers to the Prime Minister and Minister Beazley were in contact with each other. The advisers were interested partly because they realised that the size of the problem could affect Labor's chances at the next election, but also because the unexpected election victory for the ALP meant that the government was short on an agenda for reform. In addition, these particular advisers had been senior public servants in high-profile policy positions and sensed an opportunity too good to be missed.

Recollections of Labor policy advisers, March 1993

'I can remember Tom Burton, the journalist, calling me up and asking me what happened the day after the election . . . I can remember phone calls with various people—Mary Ann, maybe Meredith, certainly David Phillips—who said we must do something about long-term unemployment. They knew it was there; maybe they were getting information from the department as well as other people from Keating's office, but it had to be addressed. But because they had seen me as so involved in the research side they wanted to discuss the possibility of something happening. My involvement started with personal liaison with those people. David Phillips said, "Bring all your pictures that you have been complaining about to me and to Mary Ann and Meredith, and come and have dinner with Beazley", which I did, and they explained why long-term unemployment was an economic issue.' (Bruce Chapman)

'The Sunday after the election I thought, if Bruce Chapman is right, then we—meaning the government—are politically in deep, deep trouble. By the time of the next election, long-term unemployment would be terrible—even if the recovery came through, even if short-term unemployment lifted up, long-term unemployment would be sticking out like the proverbial sore thumb; and for a Labor government that is about the worst thing that you can get: this would be particularly bad on the Labor Government's credentials. So it is definitely Bruce's work that put this issue on the agenda and definitely a political imperative about winning an election.' (Mary Ann O'Loughlin)

'Very early on I had the sense that we had won the unwinnable election and we had gone into that election almost silent on unemployment. We had cobbled together a bit of a policy but we all

knew that it was inadequate. So I and obviously others had a very strong sense that something had to be done about that now that we had won. I rang Bruce quite early in the piece and simply said, "What have you been doing on unemployment and long-term unemployment?" I can remember trying to draw the Beveridge curve as he described it to me over the telephone. He said, "you can shift it to the left or right . . .". I then either spoke to [Mary Ann] or I had another conversation with Bruce, but that set the ball rolling. The significance of the Beveridge curve was not so much any of the theory behind it but the fact that here there was, for the first time, an argument which said there can be positive economic returns from doing something about long-term unemployment.' (David Phillips)

'My recollection is that David and I and maybe Bruce sat down and really thought through quite a bit of the strategy. We did actually think it through because we thought it was close to being overturned. We were trying at the beginning to play down the roles of Treasury and Finance. The danger was they would come in on it. So a lot of it was taking control of the processes as well as the policy.' (Mary Ann O'Loughlin)

What Chapman and others were indicating to the government through their writings and advocacy was the high potential economic costs of entrenched LTU, including the direct impact of social outlays on the budget and the *indirect* impacts on labour market efficiency, job matching, and national productivity. The Prime Minister and Employment Minister Beazley, in particular, were recognising that a reduction in LTU was essential for a productive and sustainable path out of economic recession. The economic efficiency argument gave Beazley a case for public expenditure in the short term, with expected longer-term savings. But there was still a lot about the problem that was not known.

Fortunately, after the ALP's re-election in March 1993, there was time for more deliberate consideration and the preparation of a policy program. Beazley explained the nature of the problem this way:

Immediately after the '93 election, we realised we didn't just have an employment problem, because unemployment was actually starting to come down but we had a problem that long-term unemployment was rising and we risked actually getting stuck with a large number of people permanently out of work, as they lost contact with the work-force. We judged that the best way out of that situation was to make sure that those who found themselves in that situation would be strongly encouraged to get the skills they needed. (FitzSimons 1998: 381)

As with the other three cases in this book, identifying the nature of a problem is not necessarily confined to a single stage of the policy cycle. In this case it is evident that while the problem of LTU was clearly identified in late 1992 and early 1993, its causes continued to be explored throughout 1993, culminating in the Green Paper. This exploration overlapped the policy analysis stage.

The nature and extent of unemployment and especially LTU were also under scrutiny at specific conferences, such as that held by DEET at the ANU in February 1993, and in special journal editions dedicated to the problem (e.g. the *Australian Economic Review*, no. 102, April–June 1993).

10 April 1993 (Easter Saturday) In process of arranging for Bruce Chapman to become a consultant on long-term unem- ployment issues. Met Beazley for the first time Tuesday where we took him through LTU data and related economic data . . . He asked me why we needed to do a detailed study of the LTU if we had NEWSTART. He agreed we needed to do a similar presentation to Keating now (and Willis and Dawkins) to ensure full dimensions of the problem are realised (they are more concerned about the size of the deficit at the moment).

26 April 1993 (Anzac Day) On Tuesday Beazley saw the PM on seriousness of LTU problem. Dawkins and Willis also there. Minister's office group [was set up] to progress short-term options. This week I progressed Bruce Chapman's contract to do us a LTU study. Difficulties to ensure he is clearly the best. Also refined LTU policy options paper, hopefully for the dis- cussion with D.V. and executive next week.

2 May 1993 This week was a real coup for my Economic Policy and Analysis Division; in corporate management meeting I outlined our LTU project. Next morning had first-class meeting on that issue with Volker, Hickey, Lindenmayer and Campbell on our LTU paper—for two hours a free-ranging discussion. D.V. congratulated us on the paper. Next day had Bruce C. give a seminar on the topic with D.V. there and three deputies plus three or more division heads and several Senior Executive Service officers (over 30 in total). Went extremely well. Will sign up Bruce as a consultant on LTU on Monday.

Mid-May 1993 (in London) Made £60 phone call to Chris Ryan to hear that Beazley was taking our not-well-thought- through LTU policies to Cabinet. Talked to academics here about guaranteed employment concept.

Bruce Chapman was invited to present his findings to a seminar in the Department of Employment, Education and Training in May 1993 in order to convince senior staff there, including the head of the department, Derek Volker, of the seriousness of the problem (Chapman 1993a). The seminar was also attended by advisers from key ministers' offices and from the Prime Minister's office. Soon after that presentation, DEET signed Chapman up as a full-time consultant to help determine who were the long-term employed.

ARTICULATING THE PROBLEM

> Political leaders bear a heavy burden in communicating the need for change and then creating a climate where necessary reforms are accepted. (M. Keating 1994)

After the 1993 election win, Prime Minister Keating engaged in agenda-setting activity, through, among other means, a series of press releases outlining the government's determination to address the unemployment issue.

From then on the problems of unemployment and long-term unemployment were widely discussed, with their articulation, at every opportunity, not only by ministers but also by members of Caucus and members of the CEO (see below). Comments also came from the media, academics, community groups, unions and business groups. Debates were assisted by independent policy analysis, with several groups organising public meetings and seminars on unemployment leading up to the publication of the Green Paper at the end of 1993.

Minister Beazley, in a speech to the National Press Club in June, sold the need to reduce LTU because of the economic benefits that would flow: 'high levels of long-term unemployment can actually make it more difficult to deliver low levels of inflation and unemployment in the future. This is essentially because a growing part of the unemployment pool becomes increasingly less relevant to employers' (1993: 11).

Beazley warned that because of the tendency for unemployment to 'ratchet' upwards after each recession, 'there is a real danger that the nation could develop a permanent group of unemployed people isolated from the mainstream labour market and deprived of all the social, financial and personal benefits of stable employment . . . This is a prospect which Australians cannot—and need not—accept' (p. 12).

It is a mark of the success of the government's media efforts and public messages that the phrase 'growth is required, but it is not enough' took hold. The message that LTU was costly and socially damaging was constantly echoed in the public debate and in submissions to the CEO (ACOSS 1993a; ACTU 1993; Brotherhood of St Laurence 1993a; Caucus Employment Taskforce 1993). It became a prime area of informed agreement, allowing a more focused policy search and analysis and a large measure of common purpose in the major submissions brought before the committee by interest groups.

The need for policy reform was also articulated later in the process, with DSS entering the scene with novel but relevant income support reforms as discussed below. They sold their reforms well to the CEO, meeting the committee's concerns about the work-disincentive effects of current arrangements. Later on in the White Paper process, that selling had to occur all over again to convince Treasury and Finance of the efficacy of their proposals.

> *'Treasury was not on the CEO and neither was Finance repre-sented. My recollection is that the debate on the income support measures did not finish with the Green Paper process; it went on really until the death. It was in fact when the other departments were involved in the process that there had to be a selling all over again.' (Serena Wilson)*

POLICY ANALYSIS

It should be apparent that a significant amount of analysis had already occurred in the issue identification phase of the *Working Nation* case, so that the demarcation between issue identification and policy analysis is somewhat artificial; it is nevertheless useful to treat policy analysis as a separate task or stage.

DATA AND RESEARCH

Academics played a crucial role in identifying the problem of long-term unemployment and getting it before the relevant players. This case is a good example of how a problem can be forcefully explained with timely and relevant data.

> *'We drew very heavily on the literature and research that had already been done over a very long time, particularly by Bruce Chapman and Bob Gregory. That research was much more impor-tant than the contribution of individuals wandering around the corridors of power.' (Michael Keating)*

Once the taskforce of officials was formed late in May 1993, early action was required by its expert staff to help the CEO identify and fill the gaps in the information needed for policy formulation. For example, when the CEO began its work in June 1993, basic information had to be compiled on the nature and composition of long-term unemployment. Although there was a very useful and recent summary of the evaluation of labour market programs (Jarvie and McKay 1993), there was no major synthesis of Australian evaluation evidence.

> **6 June 1993** This week we did an outline of a discussion paper to show Mike K. He had already done his . . . The main difference was his chapter on 'the importance of economic growth'. I don't see a problem with that and said I agree so long as we can make it consistent with my wanting to emphasise the need to ensure everyone who wants a job, can get one—Layard's approach (Swedish model). Economists may well buy it because it leads to reduced inflation and reduced pressure on real wages.
>
> Accomplishments this week, apart from on staffing and the outline, were several notes of advice to Mike K. with results, e.g. on how to use the Caucus Committee (mainly on consultations starting soon); and how to amend Chapman consultancy (concentrating on financing side in his interim report—after Budget). Made successful deal with ABS and contact with EPAC and DIR; and finding out which academics to bring out. Can't get Layard . . .

An immediate search, enlisting the substantial involvement of the ABS, was undertaken for relevant data and studies. DSS and DEET were mined for administrative and research data that could be used to reflect on the nature of the unemployment pool and the dynamics of long-term unemployment. Current writings were searched and used (e.g. Argy 1993). To help it in its search the taskforce set up a data subcommittee.

Processes were set up to gain information in areas where there were gaps, with many members of the CEO contributing to workshops on specific issues in their areas of expertise. A one-day workshop, for example, was held with several experts on what turned out to be a most significant area of disagreement (see below): the extent to which government intervention to assist the LTU would reduce the unemployment rate. External advice was also sought to fill several identified gaps in understanding, including new research and papers on key issues by a number of experts and consultants (ACOSS 1993b; Brotherhood of St Laurence 1993b; Chapman 1993a; National Institute of Labour Studies 1993; Purdon 1993).

Some areas could not be explored further. Guiding principles in deciding which to explore were the expected relevance of information to policy questions, and whether data could be gathered to a timetable that would allow its inclusion in the Green Paper published in December 1993 or in the subsequent White Paper policy process culminating in the Budget in May 1994. For example, the lack of Australian studies establishing the economic impacts of labour market programs was identified but could not be remedied within the required time. This became the focus of a major DEET study later (1995), as part of the evaluation of *Working Nation*.

The Green Paper was built on extensive use of Australian and overseas evaluation evidence. Evaluations of labour market programs became all the more important once it was recognised that growth alone would not solve the problem of LTU; the evidence showed that labour market programs could be effective in reducing it. In particular, subsidised employment was found to increase measurably the flow of LTU people into jobs. Without this evidence, the Job Compact (the centrepiece of the *Working Nation* labour market measures) could not have gained serious consideration (see Jarvie and Stuart 1994).

In some cases, therefore, the policy context determined which aspects of evaluation became important. In other cases, evaluation data highlighted further policy problems (see below). For example, an evaluation of the delivery of the NEWSTART program indicated a need for overhaul of client service delivery, while an evaluation of the community-based Skill Share program pointed to the potential of non-government providers to deliver flexible services to unemployed people (see Jarvie and Stuart 1994).

The work of the CEO and its taskforce was greatly assisted by a preceding period of vigorous program evaluation in DEET, and a commitment to publish information on performance. These not only contributed crucial information to the Green Paper but, arguably, prepared the ground in the community for a more informed debate.

While the taskforce was busy collecting and coordinating relevant facts and figures as well as argument, a lot of groundwork was also going on in departments. A good example of this was the work undertaken in DSS, especially by Jocelyn Pech, who was put off line for three months to research the position of the wives of unemployed men and make that research relevant to the CEO's deliberations.

KEY POLICY QUESTIONS

A comprehensive approach to policy development often involves an extensive process to canvass areas of potential disagreement before possible solutions are selected. This was certainly so in this case; for example, wider community views were gained on key issues through consultation.

There were, however, constraints on what issues of contention were examined and what resulting options were proposed. An obvious consideration was to ensure that what was analysed was consistent with the government's philosophical framework and its values. For example, deregulation of the labour market was less likely to arise as an issue under a Labor than under a Liberal government at this time. Also apparently obvious and a legitimate constraint were the terms of reference to which the CEO was working. These reflected boundaries within which the government, attempting to balance competing policy demands, wanted the CEO to operate. As Kenyon (1994: 39) notes, 'the Committee was required to focus entirely on the labour market within a strict fiscal constraint'. This arguably curtailed its consideration of the option of a larger increase in funding for labour market programs and public sector job creation (Quiggin 1993: 42).

Within those parameters, a number of key issues arose, not only during the analysis stage but also beyond the period of formal consultation and into 1994. Unlike the child support case where key questions were resolved by ministers early on followed by consultation on secondary issues, in this case contentious issues were put into the public arena through formal consultations, for example:

- how to fund the initiatives
- the nature of a training wage for younger people
- the extent to which the Commonwealth Employment Service (CES) should be subjected to competition
- work disincentives in the social security system and how to handle replacement rates
- the extent to which labour market intervention would lead to reduced unemployment (the Beveridge debate).

Two questions that appeared throughout the process but were never quite resolved were whether the focus of labour market programs should be on the shorter or longer term and what the emphasis should be between training the long-term unemployed and immediately putting these people into jobs if that opportunity arose.

The issues of funding and the training wage were the most sensitive politically and in the broader community. It is not surprising that the CEO left these two issues open in its Green Paper. It is perhaps ironic that the key issue in public debate became that of the source of funding—the heavily political issue of a special-purpose tax or 'jobs levy'. This was positive in that it focused a debate on

whether the community as broadly defined was prepared to participate in a solution, but it perhaps detracted from the debate in other
policy areas.

The CEO was aware of ACTU concerns that any training wage
might undermine award wage minimums and could lead to displace-
ment of workers. The ACTU was keen to see that labour market
programs, especially those involving training for young people,
included accreditation arrangements. The nature of training wage
arrangements was therefore going to be an inevitable point of discussion between ministers and the ACTU. All the Green Paper could do
was to present the arguments. Later on in the White Paper process,
the issue of the training wage was the most sensitive, with negotiations
still to be completed at the time the White Paper was released.

Problems with lack of responsiveness to client needs by the CES,
widely perceived to be due to its monopoly position in placing
unemployed people, arose as an issue on many occasions in consultation before and after the formal consultation process. These
problems were recognised in the Green Paper.

The issue of work incentives for unemployed people in receipt
of income support was also a view constantly placed before the CEO,
and indicated that Australia was operating with a social security
system that largely reflected labour market features of the postwar
period—for example the norm of the full-time male breadwinner.
DSS emphasised this fact in its submission to the CEO (DSS 1993:
67). This gave an additional push to the income support measures
under consideration and more strongly linked the improvement of
work incentives to increased obligations on unemployed people to
take up job offers under the Job Compact.

Finally, a purely technical but politically significant relationship
became a contentious issue among economists inside and outside the
CEO: the extent to which government intervention through labour
market programs—and particularly through a Job Compact for the
LTU—would reduce overall levels of unemployment. The debate
centred around the nature of the 'Beveridge curve', which showed
how unemployment and the vacancy rate were related. A day of
intense technical debate took place between Treasury and Finance
officers on the one hand and labour market experts Professor Barry
Hughes (of the CEO) and Bruce Chapman on the other, the former
arguing that the proposed level of intervention would lead to a
0.5 per cent drop in unemployment, the latter that it would lead to
a 1 per cent drop. The figure chosen was what would be used in
estimating the net budget cost of intervention. In the end, a compromise was struck at 0.75 per cent, which was expected to lead to

a neutral budget outcome. (Later work substantiated this as a realistic figure; see Piggott and Chapman 1995.)

> *'This [Beveridge Curve discussion] was all conducted behind the scenes, behind the CEO. I guess this partly relates to the fact that this issue was quite technical, and the members of the CEO didn't necessarily want to get bogged down in all of this.*
>
> *'In terms of the relevance of research to the policy process, this was a critical example I think. Things would have gone quite differently if we had not had the technical expertise to present these arguments, and if Treasury had had the superior expertise to destroy our arguments. It was a very academic exercise but behind this, politics and ideology were critical.'*
> *(Bruce Chapman)*

Research and analytical processes, together with the wide canvassing of views and a thoughtful set of institutional arrangements, led to policy ideas in the Green Paper that were radical, largely defensible, and had a measure of community support.

PROPOSALS AND OPTIONS

22 August 1993 Monday a.m. had significant meeting in D.V.'s office at DEET with Mary Ann, Bruce, David Phillips, Peter Grant and Stephen Moore (EPAD). Received late Thursday document on policy proposals including a guarantee of employment (and training) for the LTU. Bruce's and my idea. Strategically sold to (and now owned by) Derek. Basically going the right way. Now to sell to others.

5 September 1993 Tuesday was a CEO meeting. The result was very good in that the CEO has now focused on its policy framework including the job guarantee, at least as a serious option if it can be shown to be feasible. So our (Bruce's and mine and then Dave Phillips') careful strategy of getting its acceptance to this stage by ensuring Derek Volker took ownership of it has worked.

   . . . Thursday a.m. I went to see Beazley with M.K. and D.V. and Mary Ann with Dave P. present about outcomes of CEO meeting. Did note (at last minute) for M.K. on outcomes but he chose (wisely) to summarise where the CEO was coming out on policy. It was an excellent discussion . . . but then we turned to the timing of the release of the discussion paper. M.K. wanted to delay release until January so he could put his mark on it. Mary Ann and Beazley indicated that the PM needed a mid-December release date—before PM went over-seas. Discussion turned to how to complete a quality paper as M.K. said he was not available to concentrate on writing until end December. What about bringing in academics, said Beazley, and other suggestions. M.K. and I said it was not a matter of numbers of people but their quality . . .

I have learned heaps (and still am) from M.K.'s style. He is incredibly focused on what he wants to achieve.

3 October 1993 The PM came to the CEO meeting at midday. Good session. We had clearly got message across for something to assist LTU as well as economic growth and this was reflected in his answer to a Dorothy Dixer that afternoon.

CEO meeting was very successful. Committee members left it knowing they had a solid policy response in the form of a job guarantee but also innovative social security arrangements more in tune with the time. Lynelle Briggs's troops at DSS have done well on this one. Now down to writing it all up.

13 November 1993 It was clear that Derek Volker and Mike Keating had got together before the meeting and agreed on, at least, not using the word 'competition' in relation to the CES.

27 November 1993 Had several meetings with M.K. since his return from Seattle 6.45 a.m. Wednesday. He had asked for a bundle of our stuff, and got a big bundle on his return. I saw him 5 p.m. that day for almost two hours after he had read it all. Amazing. Each night after that I prepared several papers for him, e.g. pamphlet, overview, various chapters [revised], consultation arrangements etc. This takes more time than if I was serving a minister direct, but it does add value.

The Green Paper set out a general strategy for restoring full employment, consistent with its terms of reference. Michael Keating's preface to that document stated:

> Within that strategy, the Committee [the CEO] has presented a range of ideas for better assisting unemployed persons, and particularly those who are long-term unemployed back into work. The Committee has no fixed views on specific options at this stage, although it does believe that a substantial increase in assistance, as well as improved economic growth, will be necessary to restore full employment. (1994: xiii)

The paper took a two-pronged approach: 'the necessary first step towards full employment is to maximise sustainable economic growth' and the second step 'is to take specific government action to reduce the numbers of long-term unemployed people'. Two specific proposals were a Job Compact 'between people who have been unemployed for a long period of time, the Commonwealth Government and, more broadly, the Australian community'; and complementary income support reforms, which involved 'a fundamental restructuring of the income support system to match the major changes in the Australian labour market and in society'.

Specific options for discussion—as distinct from proposals—arose in the Green Paper in many places, for example on how to improve on the operations of the CES and on alternative ways of raising revenue, such as from a jobs levy. There were also several proposals for reforming education and training arrangements, such as a lifetime training entitlement, training bonds, a training wage, and increased entry training places for school leavers. An example of the rigour of the paper's analysis around a key proposal can be taken from the chapter 'Exploring the Job Compact'. An example of the comprehensiveness of analysis of a set of options, with careful assessment of pros and cons, can be found in the chapter 'Delivery of Labour Market Assistance', and especially the role of the CES.

Edwards and Stuart (1998: 11, 13) suggest that the large range of issues and alternatives considered by the CEO explains the widespread support for the Job Compact proposal and the limited subsequent debate over the effectiveness and desirability of labour market programs.

Compared with previous government initiatives for reducing unemployment, the Green and White Papers, in considering the problem and options for its solution, reflected a most comprehensive policy analysis process (Cockfield and Prasser 1997). Having said that, however, policy analysts did not consider in any depth certain alternatives outside the government's philosophical framework, such as the concept of work-sharing (see below).

It could be argued that the political and policy priorities of the government constrained or directed the CEO. For example, the government's ties to the union movement affected its consideration of options and the way in which negotiation proceeded; it had to take into account the unions' sensitivity to the notion of reciprocal obligation and the tightening of work tests (Lewis 1994: 12; Singleton 1994: 104). Similarly, the existence of concerns about 'dole bludgers' in certain sections of the population could be seen as the reason for including the policy of reciprocal obligation, rather than a recognition of the proven impact of strict work tests and eligibility requirements on reducing unemployment (Quiggin and Langmore 1994: 42).

The point here is that governments are elected on an understanding of having a particular set of values and directions; options developed by public servants need to be consistent with them. Any criticism that the process did not consider a wide enough range of options needs to be viewed in this context.

POLITICAL OPPORTUNISM—INCOME SUPPORT EXAMPLE

> '. . . the "less tangible" aspects of the process made the differ-
> ence. People's personal connections and networks, timing and the
> ability to put a particular rhetorical spin on proposals which reso-
> nated with key players in government were very important.'
> (Serena Wilson interview, in Howard 1998: 77)

A good example of a proposal that could be fitted with the government's values and directions but which was also generated by a set of issues not immediately related to assisting the long-term unemployed was that which emerged in the process of producing the Green Paper from DSS.

In response to the inception of the Green Paper process, senior members of DSS Social Policy Division produced a submission to the CEO in September 1993. It was an excellent example of a differing emphasis in its objectives and values as well as being a politically realistic document for policy reform. It related to the concerns of the CEO about work disincentive effects and the issue of high replacement rates, but it also met the department's own concerns that pensions and benefits might be reduced to meet this problem rather than alternative solutions supported. Another important objective of those in DSS was to ensure more independent treatment of women in the social security system, part of a long-term agenda waiting for the right opportunity. One DSS officer described how the desired income support reform was put on the agenda as part of *Working Nation*:

> I think in *Working Nation* the policy view on income support did
> come out of the Social Security Portfolio. We certainly thought that
> the income test was too punitive. You have to have the hard work
> done in terms of policy development. Then you wait for an opportu-
> nity to arise to get the policy on the agenda and implemented. It
> took us many years to get the opportunity to change the system. Gov-
> ernments don't run up to us and say 'where can we spend
> two-hundred million?' every day. *Working Nation* was this opportunity.
> (Howard 1998: 106)

The DSS proposals succeeded at this time when other similar attempts had failed (see Myers 1977; Cass 1998) because they reflected a sophisticated appreciation of political realities as well as occurring in more favourable economic and electoral circumstances.

> *'The Social Security [set of] changes that came in from left field were not in the Terms of Reference and yet they were one of the most important changes. The bureaucracy cleverly used the opportunity to get the changes through.' (Bruce Chapman)*

Although the underlying motives of the advocates of the reform were equity and social justice in the income support system as much as efficiency, they appealed to the CEO because they produced what was a rational approach to reducing the social costs of unemployment. It is interesting to note that while the income security proposals would reduce the burden of unemployment and the degree of hardship faced by couples who were both unemployed, income support changes were not significant in the CEO's terms of reference. But given Michael Keating's partiality to the measures, he effectively widened those terms of reference and so, through an iterative process, the measures became part of the Green Paper recommendations.

> **19 December 1993** This chapter is over. What a relief! A great week, apart from stress on release day. Tuesday p.m. we briefed SPC [Social Policy Committee] of Cabinet (and any other minister who wanted to come). Interesting was Dawkins' focus on process. Once Mike Keating had worked out what process he wanted (Steering Committee of relevant secretaries chaired by him) and working groups reporting to it (run by the taskforce in most cases), he did not seem to be concerned about the breadth of working parties.

CONSULTATION

The Green Paper set the following questions for its consultation with the Australian community

- How do we get from high to low unemployment?
- If you agree that economic growth must play a major role, are we prepared to make the choices necessary to speed up growth?
- Do we want to change, or are we prepared to live with high unemployment? In other words, how important to you is sharing the burden—a 'fair go for all'?

- Will the Job Compact scheme achieve its purpose of ensuring the 'job readiness' of long-term unemployed people and is it a reasonable basis for a comprehensive system of reciprocal obligations on the individual, governments, the industry partners and the community?
- What role do you see for the CES and others involved in helping the unemployed?
- How should the social security system be changed to fit better with today's labour market and changed social attitudes?
- How should extra assistance to the unemployed be funded?
- Should long-term unemployed people accept
  - a training wage while on a Government program?
  - any reasonable job and program place when offered?

Source: Abridged version of questions for the Australian community (CEO 1993: 15)

As can be ascertained from previous sections, throughout the period of the CEO's deliberations, almost constant informal consultations took place, involving either the committee members directly or the taskforce that served them. In addition, the CEO made strong efforts to undertake more formal and bilateral consultations after the release of the Green Paper, and to canvass a wide range of submissions and views through national advertisements and through personal and professional contacts. As well as that, the special Caucus Employment Taskforce, co-chaired by Swan and Sawford, busied themselves with consultations prior to the release of the Green Paper. Swan and members of his taskforce also sat in on some of the CEO's consultative meetings.

The formal and Australia-wide consultation process occurred in mid-January following the release of the Green Paper at the end of 1983 and after policy analysis had occurred. In this sense, the positioning of the consultation stage in the policy cycle between policy analysis and deciding on policy is descriptively accurate in the case of *Working Nation*.

The formal consultation process consisted of three elements:

- a toll-free hotline (receiving 340 calls)
- 1400 written submissions
- 430 face-to-face meetings.

The outcomes of public consultations were reported in a document released by the CEO. That document reported 'general community support for the overall strategy . . . in particular, the need for both a high growth strategy and measures to assist the long-term unemployed' (1994: 2). The main area of controversy was the option of a jobs levy, to which there was widespread opposition.

Stilwell (1994: 122) has suggested that the consultation process 'seemed more like a public testing of the water . . . This is a limited conception of what community consultation can be.' There may have been an element of this, to ensure a perception of wide consultation. But despite strong community support for the concept of 'work-sharing' at times of high unemployment, this support did not sway the CEO or the government since that proposal would have compromised its central objective of pursuing economic growth.

> The Committee found that, while job-sharing and reduced working hours may in some cases increase employment in the short term, they lead to a poorer long-term employment result, primarily because they lower overall productivity levels, and therefore per capita incomes. If the community generally was prepared to accept and adjust to the consequent loss of income these approaches could be viable. The risk is, however, that people would resist the reduction in living standards, adding to inflationary pressures, which could in turn reduce the total output and hours of employment available to be shared. (Ministerial question-and-answer brief for the Green Paper on Employment Opportunities 1994: 3)

The consultation process and public debate did, however, add substantially to the development of policy. The community, for example, showed a strong attachment to putting the concept of 'reciprocal obligation' into practice, and for political reasons as much as any other, this was incorporated into the proposals.

The consultation process highlighted a number of concerns that were addressed later in the White Paper. Many submissions identified the potential incentive problems associated with the design of the income support system. The role of the CES and the extent to which it met the needs of its clients—the unemployed and the employers— also came under scrutiny. As a result of the consultation process, more flexibility was introduced into the way in which the LTU were to be serviced, including increasing the degree of competition the CES faced in providing case management to them. Employers voiced concerns about hiring LTU people who were relatively untrained and unsupported, and this helped mould a more explicit link between program delivery and the Job Compact. This also led to a closer drawing together of the Job Compact and case management as a form of client training assistance (Edwards and Stuart 1998: 14). Consultation influenced the subsequent setting up of regional employment committees so that labour market programs could be more closely integrated with the wider economic development process.

> *16 April 1994* On Friday there was an important meeting of the Ad Hoc Committee on Simon Crean's submission. We cannot really determine the emphasis of the White Paper until we have the result on the training wage.
>
> *2 May 1994* Great debate about the title [of the White Paper]. Mary Ann apparently rang the PM objecting to 'Nation to Work' as anti-women and militaristic and therefore has become 'Working Nation' . . .

MOVING TOWARDS DECISIONS

> *7 May 1994* In to work by 6 a.m. Monday to collect the draft that the Prime Minister's Office worked on overnight . . . coordinated departmental comments on it from 7 a.m. and then rang PMO. They had just received the PM's comments and realised some changes to make, apart from our own . . . Raced copy to PMO 11 a.m. because AGPS deadline had been 9 a.m. But, by the hour, I was told a new version to see was to be delayed. Fed up by 3 p.m. so went for a swim.

As noted in Chapter 1 and in Bridgman and Davis (1998), the Cabinet is the official forum for final policy debates and decisions in the Australian political system.

The key Cabinet committee for overseeing the White Paper measures met many times between February and the budget in May. Ministers were asked to refine policy within guidelines set collectively by the Ad Hoc Committee of Ministers and according to a 'dollar envelope'. The setting of a budget constraint for key components of the policy package led to further evaluation and priority-setting by ministers and their portfolios. There was an intense effort within and across portfolios to develop the most equitable and effective policy for the given envelope.

In the development of the Job Compact concept, in particular, costing was extremely technical and time-consuming, requiring consideration of difficult interactions between policy and the dynamics of unemployment and long-term unemployment over time. While costing became an intense preoccupation, to specify and cost all options was clearly not possible, so an initial memorandum attempted to offer ministers choice points that would narrow the options.

One of the most difficult issues ministers had to confront was the nature of the training wage and subsidy rates for employers. In fact so difficult were the negotiations with the ACTU, that the White Paper could only refer to in-principle agreement, which awaited endorsement from the ACTU executive, before employers were consulted. The training wage rates had to be announced after the Budget (P. Keating 1994: 122).

In the context of an emphasis on economic growth, Cabinet decided to adopt the following initiatives, reforms and spending proposals.

Labour market programs and training initiatives

- the *Job Compact*, a subsidised job for those unemployed eighteen months or more based on the principle of reciprocal obligation
- increased *targeting of labour market assistance* to an individual and comprehensive *case management* for the long-term unemployed
- *reformed delivery of labour market services* such as the introduction of contracting out a portion of employment placement services to the private sector with an overseeing regulatory body
- a *Youth Training Initiative*, which increased funding for labour market program assistance to those under 18 and the transfer of Job Search Allowance recipients to a *Youth Training Allowance*, which imposed greater obligations on the young to seek work and harsher penalties for not engaging in required activities
- A *National Training Wage* for unemployed people and those receiving recognised training with significant incentives to participate for both employees and employers.

These proposals had a projected cost of $2.1 billion in 1995/96.

Social security reforms

At a cost of $280 million in 1995/96 (subject to some offsetting savings), Cabinet decided to reduce the withdrawal rate for the income test on income support and separate entitlements and income tests for partners on unemployment income support. The changes introduced a *Parenting Allowance* for partners intending to engage in the full-time care of dependants, replacing a number of dependency-based payments. Cabinet also introduced a *Partner Allowance* for partners of unemployment income support recipients (mainly women) born before 1955, allowing them to avoid the requirements of the activity test that was to be imposed on partners of the unemployed, who would now receive separate entitlements.

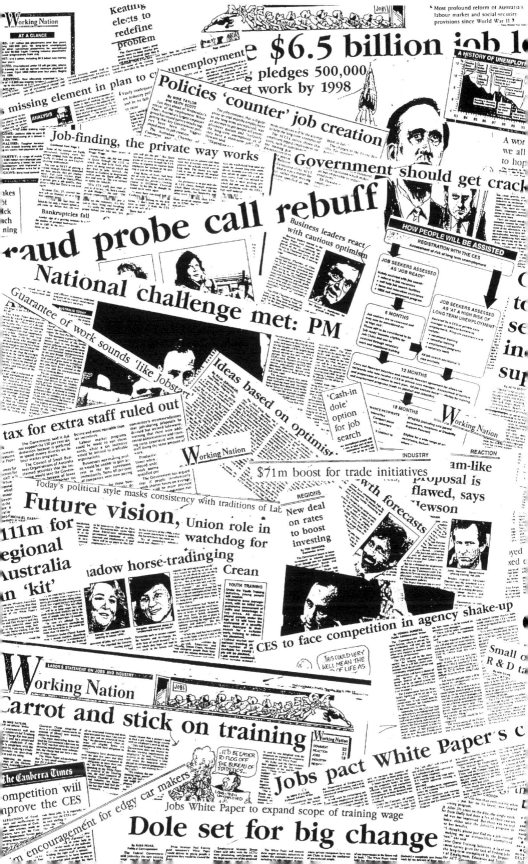

The press

The responses in newspaper editiorials on 5 May were generally positive as suggested by the following headlines: 'Tone less shrill than One Nation' (Laura Tingle in the *Australian*, p. 15); 'Genuine creativity in blueprint for the future' (Malcolm Maiden in the *Age*, p. 20) and 'Compassion and politics go together' (editorial in *Canberra Times*, p. 20).

Several journalists of the *Australian Financial Review* took a keen interest in the reforms. The *Australian Financial Review* had been consistent over the previous year in calling for more emphasis on growth measures rather than on labour market program expenditure and echoed this point again when *Working Nation* was released.

> The most important recommendation in the Green paper on long-term unemployment was growth. All the other recommendations—the Jobs Compact, reform of social security and so on—were subsidiary to the basic need to sustain very high rates of growth over the rest of the decade in order to get unemployment down to 5 per cent. (*AFR* editorial, 5 May: A3)

The concept of 'reciprocal obligation' was supported and the government was commended for a package of measures for 'helping the long-term jobless and supporting it on both equity and efficiency grounds' (ibid).

Christine Wallace in the *AFR* on 5 May predicted that the opposition would be forced to go along with the policy, given that a number of elements were 'reminiscent of Coalition policy' (p. A3). Tom Burton had followed the reform process throughout. Just before the reforms were announced, he gave readers an account of how Mary Ann O'Loughlin and others had met immediately after the election (see above p. 145), on how the CEO was set up and through to his anticipation of the contents of the budget paper ('Small post-election meeting sowed seeds of a wide strategy', *AFR*, 3 May 1994: 5).

The *Australian* was also positive. Its editorial the day after the release of the White Paper commended the government for rejecting 'hare-brained schemes' and congratulated it on its 'clever thinking about disincentives to work' and the 'long overdue' reforms to the social security system. The *Mirror*'s appraisal was particularly positive: the proposals represented a 'worthy effort right on target' (5 May 1994).

Public reactions appear to have been helped by having key journalists following regularly and seriously the academic and other debates for the year from the formation of the CEO until the budget announcements, e.g. Mike Steketee and Alan Wood (*Australian*), Tom Burton (*AFR*), Tim Colebatch (*Age*), and Ross Gittens (*SMH*). These journalists exerted some influence over a rational debate by publicising key facts and the results of research as well as their usually positive commentary.

Regional development

A number of modifications were adopted to the taxation of relevant development and infrastructure funds, and a commitment to encouraging the formation of regional councils and groupings to plan projects and increase local input in training programs, costing approximately $50 million in 1995/96.

Industry and trade development

$160 million was allocated in 1995/96 for enhancements to tax concessions for innovation, research and development, increased funding for science research and greater resources for export promotion initiatives and incentives.

> '*I don't think there is an appreciation about just how comprehensive the whole thing was—it was very comprehensive when you look at all of it—there was trade stuff there, industry development and rural development. There was all that training. A lot of the apparatus is still there.*' (Derek Volker)

Employers' needs were largely met, and there was an especially positive reaction to retaining youth wage rates for three years. The ACTU was supportive, having been in intense negotiations with the government (which was keen to bring them on side), right up until the release of *Working Nation*. Welfare groups offered qualified support, seeing the document 'as a step in the right direction' but doubting whether the funds were sufficient to assist the LTU into work in a reasonable time. Both Left and Right of the political spectrum were broadly supportive, helped significantly by expenditure on labour market programs being accompanied by the concept of 'reciprocal obligation'.

IMPLEMENTATION

It is not possible to treat all aspects of implementation announced in the *Working Nation* budget document, given the extent of the reform. Therefore only selected stories are told about aspects of implementation that focused on difficulties experienced by DEETYA.

> *'The biggest problem [for CES staff] was the sheer volume of change they had to face over many years—the breadth and intensity of the change, together with the fact that at the same time we were downsizing. People were saying, "What the hell's going on". I must say I found it extremely difficult to convince people that something new had to be done at the same time as telling them they had to do this, this and this—there were grumbles from the union that there were just not enough resources, but we managed to meet every deadline.' (Derek Volker)*

The *Working Nation* reforms placed huge demands on DEETYA officials in terms of the scale and complexity of the changes. While implementing major parts of *Working Nation*, some of which were quite novel, existing programs and services also had to be delivered (ANAO 1996: 40). It was not surprising that the department faced many hurdles and that many criticisms were made of their implementation, particularly the lack of effective coordination with other bodies.

Crucial factors appearing to affect implementation included:

- incredibly tight timelines
- perceived inadequacy of resources in relation to delivery times
- cultural resistance from within
- heavy political imperatives in an election context
- lack of clarity in objectives.

It is important to recall that *Working Nation* was the first attempt in the world to bring a competitive framework into the delivery of labour market programs in the context of a purchaser–provider arrangement. DEETYA was having to find ways to make this happen and arguably had to be ahead of the thinking of many agencies who today could be of assistance about how to contract out services, for example the Australian National Audit Office (ANAO), the Privacy Commission or the Ombudsman.

Working Nation was released on 4 May 1994. The date set for implementing its first labour market changes was 4 July, a mere two months. Expected to be in place by then were the Job Compact, JOBSTART with new rates and features, the National Training Wage (later delayed to September) and New Work Opportunities (whose projects did not start for several months). For DEETYA, these imposed deadlines could only be met if officials focused on those parts of the package that were unavoidable and essential.

Ministers appeared to be more concerned to see policies announced than to see them properly implemented. On 4 May 1994, DEETYA state managers were brought to Canberra to hear from central staff what the budget contained for them to implement. As the presentation was about to begin, the relevant senior staff were called away by Minister Crean to brief him at Parliament House about what he should say to the media. Crean would have had no idea that his demands would interfere with the necessary briefing of state managers, and neither was he told.

Because the timing for implementation was so tight, more resources were required than would otherwise have been the case to get the necessary systems up and running. This was of great concern to the head of department, Derek Volker. He was not in a position to argue that case to his Minister or to Cabinet, and hence had to play with the 'dollar envelope' allocated to his department, which led to getting the systems development in time but at the cost of resources previously committed to implementation of labour market programs.

Many critics have questioned whether the resources allocated were enough to achieve the desired employment outcome (e.g. Sexton 1994). The implementation studies of *Working Nation* found that insufficient resources were allocated to case management and training, that the government had underestimated the demand for programs, and that higher subsidies were required to make the LTU sufficiently attractive to employers (DEETYA 1996).

> *'There was a lot of organisational change and the IT revolution going on at the same time. There were massive changes. In some respects this was a bit inconvenient. It made it all that more complicated because to try to get everything to go together at the same speed when you had union resistance was extremely difficult. We got a long way down the track, but the simple fact was it was really very difficult because a lot of the targets were [high] and the legislation was delayed.' (Derek Volker)*

There was no plan to influence staff and gain cultural or attitudinal change more favourable to the reforms. Naturally many CES officers were resistant to change, not only because their perception of problems in operation did not normally match what the public was saying in the Green Paper consultation process, but also because of the fear of the unknown new world of competition. The tight timing meant that there was quite inadequate training. To the extent that there was not total commitment to the changes from some parts of the SES, this would have exacerbated internal resistance on the ground.

The next election needed to be held in the first half of 1996. The government was therefore keen to see results quickly and wanted to work on that rather than change attitudes within the organisation. This led to early announcement of schemes such as traineeships before all the detailed work could be done and departmental commitment obtained. The government was also keen to get publicity about placing unemployed people in programs since that was a lot easier than getting actual job outcomes for these people. Political factors were also at work in an attempt to marry the 'green' agenda with labour market programs. The government was keen at this period to buy the green vote.

'You can't ignore the pressures coming from the outside on implementation processes rather than the reinforcement of the objectives of reform. For example, there was political pressure to get people into traineeships, New Work Opportunities and case management. In fact there was a significant shift to New Work Opportunities. Later the pressure to deliver was enormous. Derek Volker faced this pressure from the Minister and the Prime Minister. The pressure was on to fill traineeships (which were hard to fill), New Work Opportunities (used far too often) and the purpose was to get people into the programs rather than into employment.

'What went wrong in implementing Working Nation *was that we lost the focus on the individual and ended up focusing on labour market programs and channelling people through them. What did emerge eventually was a clearer idea of the characteristics of the long-term unemployed, which was then used in the development of the Job Network.' (Ian Campbell)*

'We just had to churn people because we didn't have the right sort of economic growth then. Once people came out of Job Compact places some went back to the unemployment queues . . . There wasn't the level of job creation for a given rate of economic growth as had been the case two years previously. The conceptual underpinning was that growth would absorb new entrants with enough vacancies left to take up people ready for work after completing programs. The economy could not produce sufficient jobs for the massive targets set. Even so, long-term unemployment fell sharply. In this respect Working Nation *was successful and the basis was set for many more training places.' (Derek Volker)*

Finally, there is plenty of evidence of a deviation between the original objectives of the *Working Nation* reform and the schemes that were implemented in response to it. In part this happened because, despite continuity of key bureaucratic staff, the minister responsible for implementation, Simon Crean, had not been the minister responsible for policy development and he had different priorities. Constraints of timing, resources, culture and politics also played their part.

> '*Implementation is vital. The best-conceived policy can fail if time, commitment and resources are not set aside for planning and executing the implementation process. It's fair to say, I think, that these vital tasks were unduly squeezed in the case of* Working Nation, *with only some eight weeks allowed between the release of the government's policy statement and the full implementation of the policy. It was never a simple matter to turn around a huge system such as the CES, or to equip thousands of staff around the country for changes on this sort of scale. On this occasion the challenge simply proved too great, despite the best efforts of all concerned. For the most part, delivery on the ground fell well short of the expectations and hopes of the policymakers.' (Peter Grant)*

A useful analysis of implementation that illustrates these difficulties very well is contained in a performance audit by the ANAO, 'Implementation of Competition and Case Management'. A basic finding was that at mid-1996 there were 'differing views of stakeholders on the extent to which the competition framework was to be progressed and the timeframe in which progress was to be made' (ANAO 1996: 5). Thus the initial objectives of this set of reforms were not well understood. Specifically, the ANAO found that a number of issues remained to be resolved two years after the government's decision to implement competition in case management:

- the timeframe for progressing to a competitively neutral environment
- the application of the regulatory framework to ensure consistency with a competitively neutral environment
- arrangements for monitoring and reporting functions (see below) detailed in the Act
- funding arrangements. (ANAO 1996: 7)

The ANAO presented some broad principles of implementation which arose from experience in implementing competition in case management. It suggested that additional clarification on government policy intentions might be required—perhaps a hint that this did not occur sufficiently in this case.

It is unrealistic to set the standard at 'perfect implementation' given the complexity of the proposals and the timing of implementation (compare Gunn 1978). In *Working Nation* there were a number of 'intervening links' between the policy decision and its implementation. For example, the rates for the Job Compact subsidies had to be determined on a rolling or continuing basis by observing forecasts for future demand for subsidised placements. This introduced an extra link between the formal policy adoption decision and implementation, and the possibility that problems would emerge in the forecasting of program demand.

While this section has pointed to some significant problems in the design of the *Working Nation* package, it would be premature to simply dismiss the White Paper as a poorly implemented or unimplementable set of policy proposals. In order to properly appraise the merits of its implementation, it is necessary also to consider the existing formal evaluations of the package.

EVALUATION

The *Working Nation* budget document noted that the number of jobs required to meet the government's obligations under the Job Compact was substantial, so there was 'a need for close monitoring to allow for fine tuning, including the possible changing of subsidy rates and conditions offered to employers during the phase in period' (p. 141). It went on to propose a monitoring and evaluation strategy to provide rapid feedback on the extent to which initiatives were being successfully implemented and to give longer-term assessment of the extent to which the initiatives were reducing the number of LTU.

An important aspect of the strategy was building into the package of decisions an ABS longitudinal survey of jobless people in order to monitor outcomes and, where needed, to reorient the program. This survey was conceived when the ABS was represented on the taskforce of officials which undertook the research and policy development for the CEO. It is now a rich database for researchers.

Five factors appear to have militated against a comprehensive and creditable evaluation of the *Working Nation* reform package:

- Not all aspects of the package were evaluated; in fact the *Working Nation* document only specified an evaluation strategy for labour market assistance measures, though DSS did evaluate its social security reforms. No examination was made of a key aspect of the package, a higher rate of economic growth and its impact.
- Despite heavy expenditure, which had significant implications for a wide range of stakeholders and which might have suggested

an external evaluation process involving stakeholders such as employers and unions, the formal evaluation of labour market assistance initiatives was undertaken internally under the control of DEET in the Evaluation and Monitoring Branch.

- There were methodological difficulties in evaluating the effectiveness of the reforms, difficulties well known in Australian literature on labour market programs (see Sloan 1994; Whitfield and Ross 1996).
- The Job Compact was expected to take three to four years to implement fully, but a change of government in March 1996, less than two years after its commencement, affected the direction of reform.
- The heavy hand of strategic politics surrounded the evaluation process, on both sides of politics, as indicated below.

'This is a case where the objectives did not change but the mechanism did as it evolved, for both political and bureaucratic reasons. It was less than fully satisfactory.' (Michael Keating)

In May 1995 an interdepartmental advisory committee chaired by DEET published the Working Nation 'Evaluation Strategy' and invited comments on its suggested approach to the evaluation. Before this an externally attended seminar had been held, so to that extent there was external involvement. An interim report was to be available in 1996 and a final report in 1998. This process was to include consultation with interested groups.

The first official assessment of the impact of *Working Nation* to emerge publicly was the 1995 report *Working Nation: The First Year*, authored by Simon Crean. According to Junankar and Kapuscinski (1997: 8), 'much of the analysis was superficial. Due to the nearness of the election the report provided a very positive gloss on the labour market achievements'. This evaluation did not seek or incorporate the views of relevant stakeholders such as employers or program participants.

With the change of government in March 1996, the intended evaluation process was modified. DEETYA produced a report in July 1996 but it was no longer an interim report; the planned 1998 report was abandoned.

By the time of the report, targeted employment assistance had resulted in a substantial decline in the LTU numbers. This was acknowledged in the report: 'The reduction in long-term unemployment exceeded what could have been expected on the basis of the experience of the 1980s. High numbers of labour market program places, targeted increasingly at the long-term unemployed from

1992/93 onwards, are likely to have played an important role in this' (DEETYA 1996: vii).

The report also praised aspects of the *Working Nation* approach, such as the increase in emphasis on case management and greater competition in service delivery. But it criticised the package for the disparity between the intentions of government and what the package actually contained, being overly focused on processing large numbers of participants into labour market programs and insufficiently concerned with addressing real job outcomes for individual job seekers (pp. viii–ix).

This criticism, in fact, had been made throughout 1995, especially by PM&C officials, who were also concerned at the lower than expected take-up of Job Compact people in the wage subsidy program, JOBSTART, and the consequent big underspend compared with plans on labour market programs. It appeared that case management was being grafted onto the traditional DEETYA program structure, at the expense of assessing individual needs with more customised packages.

The 1996 evaluation report found problems with the training of case managers, and tensions between contracted case managers and the CES (p. 18). Further, it suggested that the methods of payment did not provide the maximum incentive for case managers to match the LTU with sustainable employment (p. 37). As mentioned earlier, the low take-up by employers of unemployed people under JOBSTART was reflected in this report (p. x). It also noted problems with the implementation of changes to the role of the CES—staff were unclear about what was expected of them—and noted industrial action by staff.

This report provided the basis for the Howard Government's dismissal of the effectiveness of the *Working Nation* strategy and justified an alteration of policies towards the unemployed (Finn 1997: 59). It found problems that might have reflected a change of political priorities, for example that 'a job guarantee for all disadvantaged clients was not the most appropriate strategy for assisting the long-term unemployed' (p. xi) and 'the effectiveness of case management could be improved by ensuring resources are not wasted on those who are unable to benefit from assistance' (p. ix). Interestingly, when compared to what was stated in the 1995 Evaluation Strategy document, this report redefined somewhat the main *Working Nation* initiatives, in particular putting more emphasis on an early intervention strategy and on initiatives to assist employers and not mentioning reform of the way labour market assistance was to be delivered for the LTU.

> *'The funny thing about that one [the 1996 evaluation] was that I saw a draft before I left, and the results at that time*

were better than what appeared in the eventual report. What the so-called evaluation did not take into account was that there was flexibility between programs so that Area Consultative Committees (and the CES) could put together projects which took funds/places from New Work Opportunities and other programs such as LEAP, training programs and employment subsidies so that it was difficult to identify exactly what funds went to individuals and what the outcomes were.' (Derek Volker)

Because employers were not taking advantage of wage subsidies for the LTU at the rate expected, more costly and less efficient options had to be used to give the LTU work experience. PM&C argued to John Howard when he became Prime Minister that better outcomes could be achieved with some savings if there was more emphasis on the needs of individuals through case management; in any case, if the government was to achieve the savings it was committed to from labour market programs, it would need to engage in substantial restructuring and streamlining of labour market arrangements.

PM&C officials, having felt thwarted in bringing about change, especially during 1995, seized the advantage of their position with the new Prime Minister in the first half of 1996 by undertaking considerable work in the caretaker period on new policy directions, which resulted in what turned out to be an influential discussion paper, 'Rethinking Labour Market Assistance'. This paper, cleverly crafted to be in line with the new government's election document 'Pathways to Real Jobs', identified weaknesses in current arrangements and made suggestions for reform, later largely taken up. Thus evaluation processes led on to further policy changes and the introduction of the Job Network.

> *'Despite the radical and innovative nature of the changes to employment services announced by the present government in August 1996, there were in fact some significant elements of continuity with the* Working Nation *framework. One was the competitive framework for the delivery of employment services; another the focus on individual needs and personalised assistance; and another again the targeting of intensive assistance to those jobseekers most in need. Of course, there were other elements of* Working Nation *which were discarded altogether, but that simply demonstrates the incremental nature of the policy process. When it works well, policy will learn from the past, retain what is sound and discard what is not.' (Peter Grant)*

There were a number of official and non-government evaluations of the *Working Nation* (labour market programs aspect) initiatives (e.g. ANAO 1996; Finn 1997). Junankar and Kapuscinski posed the question 'Was Working Nation Working?' and found that the labour market programs did have a small positive effect on employment outcomes and opportunities for the LTU. They argued that it was a 'very valuable social experiment which was aborted for political reasons' (1997: 1).

CONCLUSIONS

It is inevitable in the assessment of policy processes that there is no counterfactual. We cannot answer whether a lesser process would have done as well, or whether a different process could have done better. However, in assessing this policy process it is essential to understand something of the scope and interrelatedness of the policy that has resulted from it.

In scope, the policy outcomes of the White Paper included industry and regional policy as well as initiatives for employment, training, service delivery and income security. *Working Nation* provided a comprehensive strategy to boost employment growth, increase skills formation in the workforce, and ensure that long-term unemployed people are not left behind during the economic recovery Australia had entered.

> *'I would have thought that, at least conceptually, this was a classic policy model: the Green Paper, the White Paper, the whole thing, implementation built in and then evaluation on a scale that I think was unprecedented in Australia.' (Derek Volker)*

There were strong relationships between the parts of this policy package. For example, a major impediment to any proposal to reduce wages for unemployed people was the narrow gap that existed between existing low-award wages and benefit levels for couples. It was also recognised that this, together with the dollar-for-dollar withdrawal of income under the income test, was inimical to work incentives for beneficiaries. Workers could not be compelled to enter training employment if they suffered a reduction in income as a result.

This set of linked policies is interesting because it crossed port-folios and required a degree of analysis and coordination not typical of internal departmental processes. The important thing to consider here is the ambitious attempt and largely successful result in obtaining a whole-of-government approach to major and complex reform.

The cross-portfolio nature of the policy put a very high premium on coordination mechanisms to ensure this whole-of-government approach. It is unlikely that a less coordinated process, or one that was internal to government or to line departments, would have resulted in a policy package that was so fundamentally different from what had been.

The White Paper, though it may not have fully satisfied the hopes of all commentators, was well received in the community. Especially notable was the 'yes, but' response from areas usually quite divided—employer groups, unions, and the community sector. The problem definition that was undertaken led to a measure of agreement on ends, and the Green Paper and consultations helped to build a fair degree of agreement on the policy means.

Although the government may have wanted to be seen to be doing something about unemployment, this is not necessarily inconsistent with actually seeking and implementing an effective policy response to the issue. It seems reasonable to conclude that the changes to training and labour market programs under *Working Nation* did have some positive effect on the situation of the unemployed. But it is important to recognise that in these cases the social policy process was not necessarily driven by objective definitions of the problem or a sequential procedure, but instead progressed through an iterative process in which decision-makers and policy advocates both responded to and attempted to modify the policy environment by influencing the community's understanding of the nature of the issue.

In *Working Nation* it can be argued that developments in the economic, political and social environment over an extended period created pressure for reform and also affected the nature and timing of those reforms. Furthermore, it is clear that the specific institutional characteristics of the Australian government's system of providing assistance to the unemployed encouraged decision-makers to try to alter the existing policy arrangements in particular ways.

This case has shown that stages in the policy development framework do not follow a particular sequence. In fact the process in moving to *Working Nation* suggests that the social policy process is susceptible at times to considerable overlap of the stages of the policy framework. There are many examples of this, such as continuous consultation, the unearthing of relevant pieces of data throughout, the policy idea of a jobs levy being pursued early in the process, and the overlap between identifying issues for resolution and the consult-ation process. Nevertheless, it is fair to say that good policy processes were followed in this case to the point of decision, while implemen-tation and evaluation left much to be desired.

The *Working Nation* case also suggests that there is an important sense in which the policy framework is useful in descriptive terms. This relates to the tendency of governments to follow the rigour of the framework, even if only superficially or rhetorically, for political reasons. As Cockfield and Prasser note with reference to the 1994 White Paper, 'modern governments are supposed to be "rational", in the sense that their proposals are based on some theory of cause and effect, and are backed by evidence, especially in the form of numerical data. Even though decisions are made for quite obvious political reasons, governments will attempt some post hoc rational justification' (1997: 101).

This chapter has shown the relevance of both the organisational arrangements in which policy development occurs and the role of players. Especially crucial in this case was the role of academics in producing policy-relevant research on the nature and dimensions of the LTU problem. Ministers or their advisers also exercised considerable day-to-day influence to ensure the right political outcome, helped by a network based on past associations and, to a large extent, continuity of players.

Concluding observations

This concluding chapter makes some comparative observations about the four case studies in terms of movement through the stages of the policy framework. It discusses aspects of the studies which lead to suggestions for achieving better policy outcomes in the future.

FORWARDS AND BACKWARDS THROUGH THE STAGES

The general conclusion here is that in all cases, it would seem highly unlikely that the major policy changes proposed would have had a chance of being implemented without each policy stage being addressed.

IDENTIFYING THE ISSUES

Policy agendas are crowded and hence policy issues can compete intensely with each other for attention. So it is not surprising that in the cases studied it was government ministers who placed the issues on the agenda, since ultimately it is they, with their colleagues, who determine policy priorities. Even ministers can fail, in a crowded agenda, to get priority attention for their issues. In each of these cases, the ministers who did succeed not only underlined the savings to government that could be expected, at least in the longer term, but also placed each reform in a broader, usually economic, context.

Interesting commonalities across the cases can be observed in the way that later policy stages overlapped with this one. In these four cases, simple ideas were advanced that appear to have had a certain power of attraction and may have helped in the motivation to find a path through the problem to reform; without the ideas, the reform progress would probably also have stalled. For example, proposals came forward early in the policy development process for

- a 'single youth allowance' (suggested by Wilenski in 1983, four months after the ALP came to power putting youth issues high on their agenda)
- a 'child support levy' (proposed by the Family Law Council in 1985)
- a 'graduate tax' (proposed by many commentators before its acceptance by key players in 1997)
- a 'job compact' for the long-term unemployed (built from the concept of a job guarantee for the LTU that key players discussed just before the Labor Party's re-election in March 1993).

In each case, not surprisingly, the policy solution was not as originally proposed: the process of analysis and consultation, the politics involved, and the fiscal environment, led to compromises on what was for some the simple ideal solution.

'Solutions never come before the problem because that is where you get your solution from. But solutions come before the process. Sometimes the process is thought about in terms of how best to bring in a solution: what is the best way to do it.' (Bob Gregory)

POLICY ANALYSIS

A strong common feature of all cases is the amount of investment made in upfront data collection and research, which not only helps clarify the nature of the problem but is in each case important in the later direction of reform. This can be illustrated from each case, specifically showing the power of data and research in putting the problem on the agenda, if not in helping to articulate it.

- In developing AUSTUDY, the fact that research indicated there were more than thirty separate allowances being paid to Australian young people, with many in similar positions being treated differently, added considerably to the criticism of a system that was too complex to comprehend. This was on top of the other demonstrated disincentives and other deficiencies of youth allowance arrangements.

- Much timely data was unearthed at the time the issue of child maintenance came on the agenda, particularly the very useful research carried out by the AIFS. This indicated how few people were receiving child maintenance payments and, when they did, how low those payments were.
- Academics were again prominent in identifying the nature of the inequities inherent in 'free' higher education, before the introduction of HECS, by finding that since the earlier abolition of fees, the socioeconomic composition at universities had not significantly improved.
- It was labour market academics through their research findings who drew attention to the urgency of the problem of LTU, which if not tackled immediately was likely to have an adverse economic and social impact.

Three of the cases show quite clearly how the policy development process can get bogged down if decision-makers do not take the opportunity to confront key issues on which there is fundamental disagreement before options are tackled in any depth by officials.

- The OYA/SWPS discussion paper contained a range of departmental views. But the fundamental issue about the extent to which the young unemployed should have their benefits curtailed, in a fiscally constrained environment, to help other young people stay in education was not confronted (although the subject of many IDC discussions) until much later, when Dawkins took a set of key issues to Cabinet. The resulting decision provided some useful directions for bureaucrats to pursue. In this case it had become inefficient for officials to continue in circles for as long as they did in 1984, when a political decision was actually called for.
- When the Hawke Government was considering child maintenance reform in 1985, it was faced with many options— effectively a different option for each relevant departmental player on an IDC; this led nowhere. Only when Cabinet confronted a set of key issues early in 1986 and clarified their objectives—to assist sole-parent families as well as gain revenue for government—was progress made towards some in-principle decisions about the direction of reform.
- Senator Walsh placed university fees on the agenda in 1985, essentially as a savings measure, although he was keen to get rid of what he regarded as 'middle-class welfare' where the well-off benefited from free university attendance. But his option (or

options) had not confronted broader and equally significant issues, such as ensuring an expansion in the number of places in the higher education system, and so he did not get the reforms he wanted. The subsequent Wran Committee ensured that it had key issues to resolve, early on its agenda.

These three cases, as well as that of *Working Nation*, all involved both efficiency and equity objectives which, given fiscal constraints, did lead to sometimes intractable trade-offs. In other words, efficiency in the policy development process requires a judgment, as well as the opportunity, to take an issue out of the hands of officials and seek an in-principle position from the politicians before further detailed work on policy options is undertaken.

CONSULTATION

The cases in this book illustrate well the potential value of Green Papers or discussion papers in the consultation process. They show how there can be both forwards and backwards movement as the consultation process identifies issues and possibly other approaches that were not previously considered.

- The OYA/SWPS discussion paper was a useful focus for consultations as a wide range of issues on youth allowances were canvassed without one specific proposal. It also provided community groups with much information not otherwise obtainable.
- The Child Support discussion paper was different. It indicated to the public the in-principle decisions ministers had already reached before consultation and therefore was seeking views on more secondary, although still sensitive, issues.
- The HECS case was different again. There had been extensive consultations before the Wran Committee's deliberations, but based on a Green Paper that proposed educational reforms other than financing options. The committee did not undertake consultations, but it did receive submissions concurrently with its deliberations. Because ALP politics was so dominating in this case, consultation took place with the Labor Party on the basis of the Wran Report. The university sector was placated by consultations continuing with that sector right up to the start of the scheme.
- The Green Paper associated with the *Working Nation* proposals, like the Youth Allowances paper, was the vehicle for putting a range of issues and options in front of the public for debate, albeit within a framework consistent with existing government policies.

While formal consultation in each case occurred in what might be described as the middle of the policy development process, the form of consultation, its purpose and its implications differed. For example, in the Youth Allowances case the consultation process was much more open in terms of seeking views than in the Child Support case, where key decisions had already been taken, or even in the case of *Working Nation*, where the philosophical and economic framework of the government was clear and, for some of the participants, constraining. In all cases, however, the hearings in consultation processes led to changes in perspectives and, ultimately, a refinement of policy.

MOVING TOWARDS DECISIONS

In the cases studied in this book, the political process was crucial, especially at this stage. A common overriding constraint on ministers was the budget 'bottom line'. Although the government may have clearly specified the objectives of the exercise—through terms of reference or other means—and even though issues may have been clarified for officials, there was usually a very hard, ultimate decision which involved balancing broadly defined considerations of efficiency and equity. At times ministers used officials as surrogates to try to handle difficult political issues as if they could be resolved technically. Specifically, in these cases a balance had to be struck between opposing claims:

- encouraging young people to increase their educational participation but also ensuring adequacy of benefits to young unemployed people
- alleviating poverty of sole-parent families but raising needed revenue for government
- funding an expanding number of places in higher education but not deterring education access by more disadvantaged groups
- ensuring fiscal responsibility but outlaying on programs to assist the LTU get back into employment.

Sometimes the dilemma faced was met by a phasing-in arrangement in the reforms, for example in introducing AUSTUDY. In the case of Child Support, breaking up the scheme into two stages kept critics of the formula proposals at bay and ensured the longer-term revenues that would otherwise have been in jeopardy. In other cases, the reforms were introduced as a package, for example HECS was introduced alongside measures that enhanced AUSTUDY benefits. Assistance to the unemployed was a major but not the only part of the package of measures in *Working Nation* (regional initiatives were an important, if inexpensive, component).

While some important broad decisions can be made by Cabinet fairly quickly, some follow-up decisions about implementing those broad positions can be quite complex and can have a major bearing on how the policy is implemented. This was so in two cases in particular:

- In the Youth Allowances case, ministers decided to move towards equal rates for unemployed young people and students, but left the many smaller allowances to be examined by the bureaucracy; ministers were slow to give attention to problems these minor allowances created.
- In the case of Child Support, there was much legislative development that required detailed policy work for both stages of the scheme; policy development occurred while officials also worked on implementation arrangements for Stage 1.

IMPLEMENTATION

One of the messages of this book is how valuable it was in achieving outcomes, for those involved in developing policies, to have a knowledge of the implementation side and in the light of that to be able to assess the *feasibility* of achieving desired policy outcomes. There is a need to be mindful of what time and resources can reasonably be expected to be available between policy decision and implementation. The four cases show the damage that can be caused by lack of commitment in those implementing decisions—often the case if those people did not have influence over the policy decisions in the first place. Continuity of players across policy development and implementation clearly helps.

Two often neglected areas that can affect the success of implementation are publicity around the reforms and the processes around drafting the legislation. People working in these areas should be involved as early as possible in the policy development process.

Politicians often lose interest after the main decisions are made. This can mean that, unintentionally, what they hope to achieve does not eventuate. In the case of Child Support, not enough attention was given to the resource levels of the agency, the quality of its staff in the early years or the broader needs of non-custodial parents.

In the case of *Working Nation* and its implementation, politicians did not show as much concern as was necessary; for political, resource, timing and other reasons, as well as lack of clarity about what was to be achieved, policy moved away from delivering employment outcomes for the LTU and towards offering them training places to get them off the books. With HECS the process was simpler and therefore appeared more efficient: many of the implementation issues were canvassed while policy was being developed to ensure the feasibility of the recommendations coming from the Wran Committee to the government.

These two cases illustrate how important it is to anticipate some of the politically sensitive implementation issues before Cabinet makes important policy decisions. In these cases, however, the behavioural changes of the main stakeholders, such as the unemployed and employers, were very different in magnitude and breadth from the expected changes; the *Working Nation* exercise, to be true to its objectives, required much more overseeing by relevant politicians than in fact occurred.

EVALUATION

The cases in this book were evaluated in terms of the extent to which decisions of Cabinet were met efficiently. Some key concerns were singled out for careful monitoring:

- The main concern in AUSTUDY was to ensure an increase in participation in education by lower-income groups. This did occur, but the extent to which the AUSTUDY initiative could be said to account for that remains unresolved.
- In the case of Child Support, the two main concerns monitored were the extent to which sole-parent families received payments and at what rate and the extent of 'clawback' of revenue to government. Evaluations were extensive—external and internal— with more recent evaluations driven as much by a concern for how the scheme was administered as by concerns about the policy focus.
- The concern of some commentators on HECS was that it would deter access to higher education: this was monitored yearly by the Higher Education Council and shown to be not a concern, despite recent changes to the scheme that are more threatening to access. While evaluation was not extensive, it was focused.
- Despite the size of expenditure on *Working Nation* initiatives, evaluations were essentially internal to government, if not to DEET; as the case study showed, a change of government, soon after decisions, led to a change in objectives and hence what outcomes were to be subject to evaluation.

The character of the evaluation stage in policy development is influenced by whether and how that stage is linked, in an organisational sense, with earlier stages in policy development. For example, an evaluation of a policy may be undertaken by those who have initiated it or subsequently administer it, such as in the case of *Working Nation*, and the evaluation process may as a result be organised in such a way as to justify the original policy or minimise changes. The evaluation may also be initiated by the policy's critics and may be organised to demonstrate the need for changes.

In short, evaluation is not necessarily a neutral, technical exercise, but can be as politically charged as any of the other policy development phases. To understand the evaluation stage, it is therefore important to consider who initiated the evaluation, why, and how it is organised—specifically, who undertakes it and with what terms of reference.

The *Working Nation* case study, in particular, points to how easily politics can affect the evaluation process and its conclusions. It shows the need to have external evaluations which are as independent as possible from the government of the day. This seemed to be of benefit in the case of reviewing youth allowances by parliamentary committees and also, though to a lesser extent, in the Child Support and HECS cases.

A final comment is that past evaluations were used in the policy analysis stage of the policy framework in the cases surveyed, but to differing degrees. One extreme, for example, was the extensive prior evaluations of the effectiveness of labour market programs as crucial in determing appropriate policy directions for *Working Nation*. This led to incremental steps in policy which built on those evaluations. A stark contrast is the development of Child Support, where little relevant evaluative material was available anywhere in the world to help policy direction.

OTHER FACTORS AT PLAY

A major theme of this book is that a policy development framework can be invaluable in contributing to good policy processes, but it can be rather sterile, if not simplistic, if used on its own. The cases illustrate the importance of careful consideration of the organisational structures within which policy analysis occurs and of the careful selection of players in policy exercises. Above all, the cases have shown the paramount importance of politics in determining whether policy progresses from stage to stage and at what pace.

ORGANISATIONAL STRUCTURES

Apart from HECS, which mainly involved one portfolio, policy development in the other cases required cross-portfolio perspectives—if not a whole-of-government approach—to be understood, negotiated and brought together into coherent policy. This shows in the structural arrangements that were set up.

The Youth Allowances initiative was, for its time, an unusual exercise in cross-department coordination. The conventional IDC structure did not produce results for ministers, partly because of the very difficult nature of the trade-offs required by the various ministers' goals, but also because that structure was not conducive to results of the type and in the timeframe required by the driving minister, Dawkins. Dawkins relied little on the IDC process and much more on dealing with his ministerial colleagues, as well as Caucus. Moving the Office of Youth Affairs into the Prime Minister's department gave the bureaucracy, as well as the broader community, an important signal about the importance of youth issues and certainly placed OYA in a position better able to coordinate a cross-government approach to the issues than if it had remained in the Department of Education.

The Child Support case is an example of unusual structures instituted to bypass the IDC process, which also had not worked in this case. There was a need for structures to deal with complex and sensitive issues that affected many departments. It was unusual for the time to have a minister run a Cabinet subcommittee so tightly: to control its meeting times and agenda; to have a ministerial consultant working out of his department, heading the secretariat that supported that subcommittee; and to have officials meet regularly, not as an IDC (with the constraints that offered in the past) but as formal 'contacts' to advise the secretariat.

An even more ambitious structure was established in moving towards *Working Nation*, again to deal with a cross-departmental perspective—in this case a genuinely whole-of-government approach. The CEO consisted of departmental heads and outsiders as well as the Prime Minister's own adviser, served by a taskforce and not an IDC. The taskforce had representatives from several departments and took a problem-solving approach to the policy issues before them. It was quite unusual then, and has been since, to have a group of secretaries meet on a policy issue; it was also unusual for the time for ministers to meet as often as they did on what was to become the major initiative of the 1994/95 Budget.

These three cases show that, over time, greater sophistication occurred in establishing bureaucratic and political structures set up to deal with what were increasingly complex cross-departmental policy issues where there was a high premium placed on obtaining effective coordination mechanisms. They also point to the need to consider innovative policy development structures when the policy initiatives are themselves innovative.

The development of HECS, mainly a DEET policy issue, did not face the challenge of setting up appropriate structures for a cross-portfolio issue; instead it took into account what structures would fit the very sensitive political issues around bringing in some form of university fee arrangement. Dawkins played the politics brilliantly throughout and ably blended the process and people with political needs. His eye was on getting some form of fees regime through the ALP Conference later in the year, where the platform was clearly opposed to fees. He hand-picked a highly expert and dedicated group of bureaucrats to service a carefully selected Wran Committee, whose membership reflected both the Right and Left of his party. At the same time, in setting up a committee he could, if necessary, stay at arm's length from that committee.

All the cases relied on bureaucratic information exchange and debate taking place in venues other than the traditional IDC. This is not to say that IDCs cannot be the venue for constructive advice to ministers, but at least during the period covered by this book, and in three of its cases, because of past failures of IDCs to go beyond representing narrow sectional interests, other mechanisms such as a taskforce were relied on, in most cases alongside hand-picked bureaucrats.

What has been said to this point indicates that the four cases involved a certain type of minister, keen on reform, sophisticated in use of processes, as well as being a skilled politician. But the processes had to differ, depending on the circumstances and the seniority of the minister. For example, the Prime Minister could not afford to have the CEO come up with proposals that he then had to walk away from, whereas, although he may not have wished to do so, Dawkins could have done so with the Wran Committee's recommendations.

In each case Caucus was involved, usually through its relevant subcommittee. Both Dawkins and Howe knew the value not only of informing the Caucus committee but of attempting to educate Caucus throughout the process so that opposition would be minimised when final decisions were made. In the case of *Working Nation*, restiveness among backbenchers led to a specific consultation role being given to the Caucus Employment Taskforce. In the case of Child Support, bringing Caucus along with those reforms was seen as crucial, but in the other cases the role of Caucus could be said to be marginal.

THE PLAYERS

Attention has been drawn here to the careful selection of some of the players in the policy exercises driven by ministers. Ministers were looking for bureaucratic drivers who could work in partnership with them. When youth issues were a high priority of the Hawke Government, Susan Ryan as Minister for Education teamed up well, although only for a short time, with her Secretary, Peter Wilenski, a strong advocate for a youth allowance. John Dawkins had that same commitment to reform from his Special Adviser on Youth Allowances, as did Brian Howe in those from his department in the Maintenance Secretariat. Dawkins hand-picked his bureaucratic team from within DEET, with a committed leader in Alison Weeks and an involved division head in the department. And Paul Keating could rely on dedication and commitment to reform from his head of department, Dr Michael Keating.

> 'The interesting thing was that in the 1980s you had the growth of ministerial advisers—much stronger ministerial advisers than we had seen, as a generality, in the past.' (Vic Rogers)

Also interesting to note is the role played in each case by ministerial advisers and consultants. The extent of their ministers' reliance on them indicates the importance to the relevant minister of the reform initiatives:

- Dawkins, on becoming Minister assisting the Prime Minister on Youth Affairs, dedicated a senior adviser in his parliamentary office, Allen Mawer, to work full-time on youth issues. The result was a very close working relationship between him and the special adviser in PM&C with whom he prepared submissions for Dawkins.
- Howe, against convention, appointed a ministerial consultant to work full-time on child maintenance out of his department, and later another ministerial consultant, this time working from his parliamentary office, to oversee more detailed policy work and the legislation.
- Dawkins hired a consultant to work full-time on the Green Paper and then to assist in the HECS process. His senior adviser kept a close eye on Wran Committee activities.
- Prime Minister Keating used his staff extensively in the *Working Nation* process, including placing his senior social policy adviser on the crucial CEO to help guide the issues through to the 1994/95 Budget.

'Political opportunism' was evident in the case of *Working Nation*, in particular when a group of public servants in DSS brought forward their pet proposals. This was an example of what has been called 'policy entrepreneurship': 'Policy entrepreneurs, people who are willing to invest their resources in pushing their pet proposals or problems, are responsible not only for prompting important people to pay attention, but also for coupling solutions to problems and for coupling both problems and solutions to politics' (Kingdon 1984: 21). The group of DSS officials who had been working on a particular set of policies for some years found the right angle and right timing to have a significant influence on the income support policies contained in *Working Nation* (Howard 1998). It could be argued that these policies would have been forthcoming anyway, despite the players, but that is most unlikely in this case, since the terms of reference for the CEO did not place emphasis on social security reforms.

Academics were actively involved in each case, often coming into the bureaucracy for a short time and/or serving regularly on policy-advising committees (for example, outside lawyers in Child Support, labour market economists in Youth Allowances, and Bruce Chapman in HECS and *Working Nation*).

Informal networks of key players were especially noted in the process of putting LTU on the agenda, where key ministerial advisers, bureaucrats and academics were in constant contact through informal processes. It also occurred in other cases and was particularly beneficial in Child Support, where informal contacts with the legal profession, social welfare and women's groups were important in minimising adverse comment on the proposed reforms.

Mention should also be made of the value of continuity in the involvement of officials, politicians and other players, both through the stages of policy development as well as across reforms. That helped to build networks, but also led to a greater likelihood that original policy intentions would be translated into practice.

The final observation here is the role of the media in influencing public opinion. Some key journalist commentators (e.g. Kate Legge of the *Age*, Mike Steketee of the *Australian*, Ross Gittens of the *Sydney Morning Herald*) followed policy development throughout and were encouraged to do so by relevant ministers or their advisers. In each of the cases, the facts and logic around the reform proposals on the whole resonated with these commentators, who in turn mostly put the reforms in a positive light, or at least concurred with the need for reform.

LOOKING TOWARDS THE FUTURE

More junior-level public servants may consider, after reading through the cases, that there is little in the policy process that they can influence; and in any case it's all too hard if major reform is to be achieved, particularly given the paramount importance of 'politics'. It is true that major reform is difficult, and sometimes it has to be achieved at breakneck speed, which leaves more junior (if not senior) officials feeling as if their work life is out of control, but it is not true that influence is impossible. With constant and big doses of persistence, there are several ways of having an influence beyond playing wording exercises with colleagues:

- know the power of data and use that to advantage
- keep in touch with relevant academic research
- ask questions about what are the key issues on which agreement can be found
- encourage colleagues to take a problem-solving rather than adversarial and narrow departmental approach, especially on IDCs
- explore lateral approaches to solving problems and getting agreement on issues
- clarify policy objectives, with superiors where necessary
- be rigorous in analysis, pointing out all possible implications of options
- be aware of the need to consider implementation issues in designing policy.

There is also, of course, the opportunity provided by networking with people inside as well as outside the bureaucracy, which can also lead to useful knowledge about the broader political and economic context of reforms.

This book aims to make a contribution toward advancing bureaucratic policy processes, and to assist students of public policy to understand those processes. It is hoped that these case studies will advance theoretical and conceptual constructs about what does constitute good policy development processes and, perhaps, clarify the factors that can prevent policy initiatives from stalling.

This book ends with three practical suggestions for ensuring more efficient and effective policy development processes for governments in the future:

- introduce a *systematic approach to evaluating policy advice* and how policy is developed
- ensure that *collaborative interdepartmental structures* are set up to get interdepartmental cooperation
- nurture *links with academics* who have the capacity to be involved in policy research and policy development processes.

First, there is a strong case for introducing mechanisms to assess the value of policy development exercises—more broadly, to evaluate the policy-advising function and learn from experiences. Apart from the need for policy advisers to be accountable for their work, ministers 'have a right to know whether the policy advice they receive . . . meets standards of rigour, honesty, relevance and timeliness' (Waller 1992: 440).

The Commonwealth Government, mainly through the efforts of the Departments of PM&C and Finance, did begin this process in the first half of the 1990s, but it has since fallen into abeyance, except for some elements undertaken by the ANAO. Essentially the practice in the past was for an outside consultant with bureaucratic expertise, using internal documentation and other means, to assess the policy process according to a framework such as that adopted in this book (Edwards 1996).

Policy assessments that have been undertaken (e.g. Glenn 1993; Weller 1995) have been found to be valuable teaching resources in policy skills workshops. The use of evaluations of policy development processes in training courses has great benefit. The resulting documentation can help train officials and assist their agencies to become 'learning organisations' on policy development: officials can be alerted to potential problems and how they might be overcome, especially when complex policy work is involved (Podger 2000: 127). A side benefit is the strengthening of institutional memory.

Governments today are focusing much more on meeting the needs of clients in developing policy and delivering services, and as a result policy activity is spanning many programs, portfolios and even the whole of government. There is therefore a real need to come to grips with evaluation processes which are cross-program, cross-portfolio and even cross-government.

Suggestion two is to devise structures which can counter the all too often artificial nature of departmental divisions when it comes to good policy advice. In the case of Child Support, certain agencies, such as DSS, but also coordinating agencies, had strong interest in particular aspects of policy development; Attorney-General's was most interested in drafting legislation, and the ATO, naturally, wanted to ensure that implementation would be feasible. This point has been well made recently by the Ralph Review (1998). Understanding the perspective of other organisations and taking that into account throughout the process requires structures that maximise a systematic and cooperative approach.

IDCs do all too often thwart this process. There is a constant danger that this forum for providing advice to ministers will fall into disrepute, if not be bypassed, unless senior officials and ministers consider carefully how interdepartmental meetings are best to serve policy-makers. There is scope to turn IDCs into problem-solving rather than department-serving forums, but that requires strong leadership from senior departmental officers, if not ministers, and a clear understanding of what they expect of public servants as well as a willingness to intervene when the issues go beyond the technical into the political. More broadly, having the climate to pursue good policy processes depends on ministers understanding the part that good bureaucratic processes can play in achieving their objectives.

Finally, the case studies in this book have shown the significant role that academics can play in initiating ideas and contributing to policy analysis. It is extremely important therefore for policy advisers and policy-makers to nurture their links with academics who undertake research relevant to policy, especially when fundamental policy change is being considered. Policies analysed in this book were unlikely to have seen the light of day without the involvement of academics at different stages of policy development. Exchange needs to occur in as many ways as possible between academics and policy advisers, in the interests of both the content and processes of good public policy.

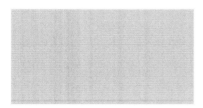

Bibliography

PREFACE

Colebatch, H. K. 1998, *Policy*, Buckingham: Oxford University Press

Edwards, M. 1992, 'Evaluating Policy Advice: A comment', *Australian Journal of Public Administration* 51(4): 447–9

Waller, M. 1992, 'Evaluating Policy Advice', *Australian Journal of Public Administration*, 51(4): 440–6

Yeatman, A. (ed.) 1998, *Activism and the Policy Process*, Sydney: Allen & Unwin

CHAPTER 1 INTRODUCING POLICY PROCESSES

Bailey, M. T. 1994, 'Do Physicists Use Case Studies?', in J. D. White and G. B. Adams (eds), *Research in Public Administration: Reflections on Theory and Practice*, London: Sage, pp. 183–96

Bridgman, P. , and G. Davis 2000, *Australian Policy Handbook*, Sydney: Allen & Unwin

Colebatch, H. K. 1998, *Policy*, Buckingham: Oxford University Press

Committee on Employment Opportunities 1993, *Restoring Full Employment: A Discussion Paper*, Canberra: AGPS

Dalton, T., M. Draper, W. Weeks and J. Wiseman 1996, *Making Social Policy in Australia: An Introduction*, Sydney: Allen & Unwin

Davis, G., J. Wanna, J. Warhurst and P. Weller 1993, *Public Policy In Australia*, Sydney: Allen & Unwin

Dror, Y. 1964, 'Muddling Through—"Science" or Inertia,' *Public Administration Review*, 24(3): 153–7

Dunleavy, P. 1995, 'Policy Disasters: Explaining the UK's Record', *Public Policy and Administration*, 10(2): 52–70

Edwards, M. 1992, 'Evaluating Policy Advice: A Comment', *Australian Journal of Public Administration*, 51(4): 447–9, reprinted as 'Politics and Judgement' in Uhr and Mackay, *Evaluating Policy Advice*, pp. 21–5

——1993, Child Support Scheme: Policy Development Processes and Practices, Mimeo, based on presentation to AIC Conference, April

——1996, Lessons from Prime Minister and Cabinet, in Uhr and Mackay, *Evaluating Policy Advice*, pp. 73–82

Gunn, L. 1978, 'Why is Implementation so Difficult', *Management Sciences in Government*, 3: 169–76

Hall, P., H. Land, R. Parker and A. Webb 1986, *Change, Choice and Conflict in Social Policy*, Hants UK: Gower Publishing Company (first published 1965)

Hawke, G. R., 1993, 'Improving Policy Advice', Institute of Policy Studies, Victoria University of Wellington, Wellington: Printing Press

Hill, M. 1997, *The Policy Process in the Modern State*, 3rd edn, London: Prentice Hall

Hogwood, B. W., and L. Gunn 1984, *Policy Analysis in the Real World*, Oxford: Oxford University Press

Howard, C. 1998, *Carrots and Sticks: A Means Testing State Changes its Mind*, honours dissertation, Griffith University

Howlett, M., and M. Ramesh 1995, *Studying Public Policy*, Toronto: Oxford University Press

Hummel, R. P. 1994, 'Stories Managers Tell: Why they are Valid as Science', in White and Adams, *Research in Public Administration*, pp. 225–45

Keating, M. 1996, 'Defining the Policy Advising Function', in Uhr and Mackay, *Evaluating Policy Advice*, pp. 61–7

Keating, P. 1994, *Working Nation: Policies and Programs*, Canberra: AGPS

Lindblom, C. E. 1959, 'The Science of "Muddling Through"', *Public Administration Review*, 19: 78–98

May, A., and A. Wildavsky (eds) 1978, *The Policy Cycle*, Beverly Hills, CA: Sage

May, P. J. 1991, 'Reconsidering Policy Design: Policies and Politics', *Journal of Public Policy*, 11(2): 187–206

Nakamura, R. 1987, 'The textbook policy process and implementation research', *Policy Studies Review*, 7: 142–54

Office of Regulation Review, 1998, *A Guide to Regulation*, 2nd edn, Commonwealth of Australia, December

Painter, M., and B. Carey 1979, *Politics Between Departments*, Brisbane: University of Queensland Press

Parsons, W. 1995, *Public Policy: An Introduction to the Theory and Practice of Policy Analysis*, Aldershot, UK: Edward Elgar

Peters, B. G., and F. K. Van Nispen 1998, *Public Policy Instruments: Evaluating the Tools of Public Administration*, Cheltenham, UK: Edward Elgar

Review of Business Taxation (Ralph Review) 1998, *A Strong Foundation: A Discussion paper, Establishing Objectives, Principles and Processes,* Canberra: AGPS

Ryan, N. 1995, 'Unravelling Conceptual Developments in Implementation Analysis', *Australian Journal of Public Administration*, 54(1): 65–80

Uhr, J., and K. Mackay (eds) 1996, *Evaluating Policy Advice*, Federalism Research Centre, ANU, and Commonwealth Department of Finance, Canberra

Weller, P. , and B. Stevens 1998, 'Evaluating Policy Advice: The Australian Experience', *Public Administration*, 76(Autumn): 579–89

White, J. D., and G. B. Adams (eds) 1994, *Research in Public Administration: Reflections on Theory and Practice*, London: Sage

CHAPTER 2 INCOME SUPPORT FOR YOUNG PEOPLE

ABS 1985, *Australia's Youth Population 1984: A Statistical Profile,* ABS, Canberra

ANOP 1984, *Young Australians Today*, Department of Sport, Recreation and Tourism, Canberra: AGPS

Baird, C., R. Gregory and F. Gruen (eds) 1981, *Youth, Employment, Education and Training*, Conference papers, Academy of Social Sciences, Centre for Economic Policy Research, Canberra: ANU Press

Bureau of Labour Market Research 1983a, *Employment and Training Programs for Young People: Analysis of Assistance in 1980–81*, Research Report No. 2, Canberra: AGPS

——1983b, *Youth Wages, Employment and the Labour Force*, Research Report No. 3, Canberra: AGPS

Chapman, B. 1992, 'Austudy: Towards a more flexible approach—An options paper', report commissioned by DEET, April, Canberra: AGPS

Dawkins, J. S. 1985, *Reform of Youth Income Support*, Press Statement, Canberra, July

Dawkins, J. S. and P. Walsh 1985, *Youth Policies in the 1985/86 Budget*, 1985/86 Budget paper No. 13, August, Canberra: AGPS

——1986, *Young Australia and the 1986/87 Budget*, Canberra: AGPS

Department of Education 1985, *Annual Report 1984–85*, Canberra: AGPS

Department of Education 1986, *Student Assistance for the Disadvantaged: Practice and Prospect*, papers delivered at seminar, December 1985, Canberra: AGPS

Department of Employment and Industrial Relations 1985, *Annual Report 1984–85*, Canberra: AGPS

Department of Prime Minister and Cabinet 1986, *Annual Report, 1985–86*, Canberra: AGPS

DEYA 1983a, *Annual Report 1982–83*

——1983b, *Youth Policies Programs and Issues: An Australian Background Paper, I*, Canberra: AGPS

——1985, Recommendation by Recommendation Responses to the OECD Review of Youth Policies in Australia (unpublished)

Edwards, M. 1984, 'Youth Allowances—Issues and Options', *Canberra Bulletin of Public Administration*, xi(2): 105–10

——1985a, 'Youth Income Support for Under Eighteen Year Olds', Welfare Rights Centre Seminar, Canberra

——1985b, 'Youth Allowances: Incentive and Reform Issues', Paper presented to the 54th ANZAAS Congress, Canberra, May, published 1985 in *Australian Journal of Social Issues*, 20(1): 35–55

——1986, 'Attainable Goals', in *Student Assistance for the Disadvantaged: Practice and Prospects*, Department of Education

Gregory R., and R. C. Duncan 1980, 'High Teenage Unemployment: the role of a typical labour supply', *Economic Record*, 56: 301–15

Gregory, R., and P. Stricker 1982, 'Youth Employment and Unemployment: the Australian Experience in the 1970s', in Baird, Gregory and Gruen, *Youth, Employment, Education and Training*

Ironmonger, D. 1983, 'Financial Incentives for Teenagers: A Sensible Structure', paper presented to the 53rd ANZAAS Congress, Western Australia, May

Hawke, R. J. L. 1985, *The Commonwealth Government's Strategy for Young People, a Statement by the Prime Minister*, Canberra: AGPS

HRSC on Employment, Education and Training 1989, 'The restless years: an inquiry into Year 12 retention rates', 2 November

——1991, 'Student financial assistance', 11 April

Kemp, D. 1999, 'An Australian Perspective', Paper presented to OECD Conference 'Preparing Youth for the 21st Century: the Policy Lessons from the Past Two Decades', Washington DC, 22–23 February

Kirby, P. 1985, *Report of the Committee of Inquiry into Labour Market Programs*, Canberra: AGPS

OECD Manpower and Social Affairs Committee 1984, *Review of Youth Policies in Australia*, November, Paris: OECD

OYA 1984, *Education Participation and Financial Incentives*, Working Paper prepared by Julie Smith, DEYA

——1985, *'Young Australia'*, *Part A, A Background to Reform*, Canberra: OYA

OYA/SWPS 1984, *Income Support for Young People*, Canberra: AGPS
Senate Employment, Education and Training References Committee 1995, 'AUSTUDY', June
TFYAA 1986, 'On the options for incorporating selected non-mainstream schemes into the common allowance structure', March
YACA 1983, *Creating Tomorrow Today*, July, Melbourne: YACA
Wilenski, P. 1983, 'Youth Policy and Youth Allowances', Paper presented to conference on Learning and Earning, Darling Downs Institute of Advanced Education, Toowoomba, Queensland, 30 June–3 July

CHAPTER 3 FROM CHILD MAINTENANCE TO CHILD SUPPORT

AIFS 1984, *The Costs of Children in Australia* (Lovering Report), August
——1990, *Who Pays for the Children?* Interim Report on Stage 1, August
——1991, *Paying for the Children, Final evaluation of Stage 1*, June
Attorney-General's Department 1984, *A Maintenance Agency for Australia: The Report of the National Maintenance Inquiry*, Canberra: AGPS
Brennan T. 1995, Address to Public Policy Program, University of Melbourne (unpublished transcript)
Bridgman, P. , and G. Davis 2000, *Australian Policy Handbook*, 2nd edn, Sydney: Allen & Unwin
Cabinet Subcommittee on Maintenance 1986, *Child Support: A Discussion Paper on Child Maintenance*, Canberra: AGPS
Clarke, D.1987, 'The tax man takes a greater role in child support—without too much discussion', *AFR*, 13 January
CSCG 1988, *Child Support: Formula for Australia*, Canberra: AGPS
——1989, *The Child Support Scheme: Progress of Stage One*, August, Canberra: AGPS
CSEAG 1990, *The Child Support Scheme: Adequacy of Child Support and Coverage of the Sole Parent Pensioner Population*, Canberra: AGPS
——1992, *Child Support in Australia: Final Report of the Evaluation of the Child Support Scheme*, 2 vols, Canberra: AGPS
DSS 1994, *Child Support Scheme:* Submission to the Joint Select Committee on Certain Family Law Issues, DSS
Edwards, M. 1986a, 'Report on Consultations on Child Support', in *Proceedings of Income Support Seminar*, Meeting of Social Welfare Administrators, December, pp. 194–201
——1986b, 'Child Support: Assessment, Collection and Enforcement Issues and Possible Directions for Reform, Child Support', Social Justice Project Conference papers, ANU, February, pp. 1–42
——1988, 'The New Face of Child Maintenance—Towards 1990', Paper presented to Bicentenary Family Law Conference, Melbourne, March

——1992, 'Evaluating Policy Advice: A Comment', *Australian Journal of Public Administration*, 51(4): 447–9

——1993, 'Child Support Scheme: policy development, processes and practices', mimeo, based on presentation to AIC Conference, April

Edwards, M., T. Harper and M. Harrison 1985, 'Child Support: Public or Private Duty?', *Australian Society*, 4(4): 18–22

FLC 1985, Family Law Council Report on Maintenance Enforcement, December (unpublished)

Fogarty, Justice J. 1986, Commentary on the paper delivered by Dr Meredith Edwards, on the Family Law Council's Proposals for Maintenance Reform, June (unpublished)

Garfinkel, I. 1979, 'Welfare Reform: a new and old view', Discussion Paper, Institute for Research and Poverty, University of Wisconsin

Harrison, M., T. Harper and M. Edwards 1984, 'Child Support: Public or Private Duty?', Paper presented to conference on Family Law in 1984, Hobart, 1984. Reproduced in abridged form in *Australian Society*, 4(4): 18–22

Holub, L. 1989 'The Child Support Agency—A New Era in Child Maintenance', Australian Public Policy Case Library, Public Policy Program in collaboration with Royal Australian Institute of Public Administration, ACT Division, ANU, October

Howe, B. 1986, 'Major Reform of the Child Support and Maintenance System', Press Release, 19 August

——1987a, Minister for Social Security, News Release, 'Government decides on new Child Support System', March

——1987b, Minister for Social Security, Press Statement, 'Government decides on new Child Support System', March

Lee Patterson & Associates 1988, Report on Public Relations Program for Stage 1, Child Support Scheme, DSS, September

McDonald, P. 1985, 'The Economic Consequences of Marital Breakdown', AIFS, Melbourne, August

——(ed.) 1986, *Settling Up: Property and Income Distribution on Divorce in Australia*, Sydney: Prentice-Hall

McDonald, P. , and R. Weston 1986, 'The Data Base for Child Support Reform', Child Support, Social Justice Project, ANU, pp. 74–86

Parliament of Australia 1994, Joint Select Committee on Certain Family Law Issues, 'Child Support Scheme: An Examination of the Operation and Effectiveness of the Scheme', Parliament of the Commonwealth of Australia, November

CHAPTER 4 PAYING FOR A UNIVERSITY EDUCATION

ALP 1988, Platform Resolutions and Rules

Anderson, D. S., and A. E. Vervoorn 1983, 'Access to Privilege: Patterns of Participation in Australian Post-Secondary Education', ANU, Canberra

Blandy, R. M. 1979, 'A Liberal Strategy for Reform of Education and Training in Australia', in Australian Commission of Inquiry into Education and Training, Education, Training and Employment Report, February

Blewett N. 1999, *A Cabinet Diary*, Kent Town, SA: Wakefield Press

Bulbeck C. 1987, 'Financing Tertiary Teaching—an income tax levy scheme', *Australian Universities Review*, 30(1): 40–1

Chapman, B. 1996a, 'The Study of Economics and Direct Involvement in Policy: The Case of the Higher Education Contribution Scheme', Bankers Trust Lecture, Bankers Trust Australia Ltd, November

——1996b, 'Conceptual Issues and the Australian Experience with Income Contingent Charges for Higher Education', ANU, August

——1998, 'Economics and Policy-making: the case of the higher education contribution scheme', *Canberra Bulletin of Public Administration*, 90 (December): 120–4

Chapman, B., and D. Smith 1995, 'The Higher Education Contribution Scheme After Five Years', *Current Affairs Bulletin*, January–February

Committee on Higher Education Funding 1988a, *Report of the Committee on Higher Education Funding* (the Wran Report), Commonwealth of Australia

——1988b, 'The Wran Report: Commentary on Public Responses', Commonwealth of Australia

CTEC 1987, Review of Efficiency and Effectiveness in Higher Education, Canberra: AGPS

Dawkins, J. S. 1987a, *The Challenge of Higher Education in Australia*, Canberra: AGPS

——1987b, *Higher Education: A Policy Discussion Paper* (Green Paper), Canberra: AGPS

——1988a, *Higher Education: A Policy Statement* (White Paper), Canberra: AGPS

——1988b, *A New Committment to Higher Education in Australia*, Canberra: AGPS

——1988c, 'Minister Calls for Comment on Wran Report', Media Release, 5 May

Friedman M. 1955, 'The Role of Government in Education', in A. Solo (ed.), *Economics and the Public Interest*, Rutgers University Press, pp. 123–44

Kingdon, J. W. 1995, *Agendas, Alternatives, and Public Policies*, 2nd edn, Boston: Harper Collins

Manning, I. 1986, 'Alternative finance for tertiary teaching', *Australian Universities Review*, 29(2): 2–8

NBEET 1992, Assessment of the Impact of the Higher Education Contribution Scheme on the Potentially Disadvantaged, Commissioned Report No.15, Canberra: AGPS

Power, C., and F. Robertson 1987, 'Effects of the Administration Charge on Participation in Higher Education by Full-Time and Part-Time students', National Institute for Labour Studies, Flinders University, September

Robertson, F., J. Sloan and N. Bardsley 1989, 'The Impact of the Higher Education Contribution Scheme (HECS) on Participation in Higher Education in Victoria and Western Australia in 1989', National Institute of Labour Studies, Flinders University, January

Walsh P. 1995, Confessions of a Failed Finance Minister, Sydney: Random House

Wells, M. C. 1987, 'Using the tax system to collect fees', Australian Universities Review, 30(2): 32–3

Wran Report, see Committee on Higher Education Funding 1988a.

CHAPTER 5 LONG-TERM UNEMPLOYMENT POLICY

ACOSS 1993a, Federal Budget Priorities 1993–1994, Submission to the Federal Government, paper No. 55, Sydney

——1993b, Report of an Investigation of Approaches, Programs and Policies for Those Most Disadvantaged in the Labour Market, Consultant's Report prepared for the Taskforce on Employment Opportunities, September

ACTU 1993, A Program Towards Full Employment: The ACTU's Program for Sustainable Employment and Jobs Growth for the 1990s and Beyond, Submission to the Committee on Employment Opportunities

ANAO 1996, Implementation of Competition in Case Management, Audit Report No. 30, 1995/96, Canberra: AGPS

Argy, F. 1993, 'An Australia that Works: A Vision to the Future. A Long-term Economic Strategy for Australia', CEDA Research Study, p. 38

Beazley, K. 1993, 'Full Employment: Vision or Illusion?', speech at National Press Club, Canberra, 30 June

Bridgman, P. , and G. Davis 2000, Australian Policy Handbook 2nd edn, Sydney: Allen & Unwin

Brotherhood of St Laurence 1993a, A Strategic Approach to Reducing Unemployment, Submission to the Committee on Employment Opportunities

——1993b, Existing but Not Living: A Research Project Canvassing the Attitudes, Expectations, Aspirations and Views of Long-Term Unemployed Australians, Consultant's Report prepared for the Taskforce on Employment Opportunities

Burton, T. 1994, 'A small post-election meeting sowed seeds of a wider strategy', *AFR*, 3 May: 5

Cass, B. 1988, *Income Support for the Unemployed in Australia: Towards a More Active System*, Canberra: AGPS

Caucus Employment Taskforce 1993, *'Growth Plus' Equals the Employment Challenge: A Positive Agenda for Change*, Submission to the Committee on Employment Opportunities

CEO 1993, *Restoring Full Employment: A Discussion Paper*, Canberra: AGPS

CEO 1994, *Report on Public Consultations,* Prime Minister and Cabinet, Canberra

Chapman, B. 1993a, 'Long Term Unemployment: Causes, Costs and Policy Responses', report to DEET, mimeograph, Canberra

——1993b, 'Long-Term Unemployment: The Dimensions of the Problem', *Australian Economic Review*, 2nd Quarter: 22–5

Chapman, B. J., P. N. Junankar and C. A. Kapuscinski 1992, 'Long Term Unemployment Projections', *Australian Bulletin of Labour*, September: 195–207

——1993, 'Long Term Unemployment', paper presented to 'Unemployment: Causes, Costs and Solutions' conference, Canberra, February

Cockfield, G., and S. Prasser 1997, 'Policy statements: visions or burdens?', in G. Singleton (ed.), *The Second Keating Government: Australian Commonwealth Administration 1993–1996*, Canberra: Institute of Public Administration Australia

DEET 1995, *Working Nation: Evaluation Strategy*, Canberra: AGPS

DEETYA 1996, *Working Nation: Evaluation of the employment, education and training elements*, Canberra: AGPS

DSS 1993, *Meeting the Challenge: Labour Market Trends and the Income Support System,* Canberra: AGPS

Edwards, J. 1996, *Keating: the inside story*, Melbourne: Penguin Books Australia

Edwards, M., and A. Stuart 1996, 'The 1994 White Paper—A Preliminary Review of a Policy Process', Proceedings of the International Conference of the Australasian Evaluation Society, *Evaluation: making performance count*, Canberra, pp. 73–82

Finn, D. 1997, *Working Nation: Welfare Reform and the Australian Job Compact for the Long Term Unemployed*, Sydney: ACOSS

FitzSimons, P. 1998, *Beazley: A Biography*, Sydney: HarperCollins

Fraser, B. W. 1998, 'Aspects of Growth', in Reserve Bank of Australia, *Collected Speeches: B. W. Fraser, Governor Reserve Bank of Australia. 1989–1996*, vol.1, RBA, pp 253–64, Sydney

Grant, P. 1998, 'Choice and Competition in Employment Placement Services', *Canberra Bulletin of Public Administration*, 88, May, pp. 77–82

Jarvie, W., and R. McKay 1993, Perspectives on DEET Labour Market

Programs, EMB Report, 1/93, Economic Policy and Analysis Division, DEET

Jarvie, W., and A. Stuart 1994, 'The use of Evaluation in "Working Nation"', Proceedings of the International Conference of the Australasian Evaluation Society, *Evaluation: Making Performance Count*, Canberra, pp. 167 76

Junankar, P. N., and C. A. Kapuscinski 1997, Was Working Nation Working?, unpublished discussion paper, ANU Public Policy Program, Canberra

Keating, M. 1993, 'Emerging Trends in The Labour Market', Paper presented to Conference on Social Security Policy, Canberra, 4–5 November

Keating, P. 1993, 'The revolution in our economy must continue', *SMH*, 10 February

——1994, *Working Nation*, Canberra: AGPS

Kenyon, P. 1994, 'Restoring Full Employment: Backing An Outsider', *Australian Economic Review*, 1, 1st Quarter: 31–46

Layard, R., S. Nickell and R. Jackman 1991, *Unemployment, Macro-economic Performance and the Labour Market*, Oxford: Oxford University Press

Lewis, P. E. T. 1994, 'Long-term Unemployment: The Role of Wage Adjustments', *Economic and Labour Relations Review*, 5(1): 11–20

Myers, D. 1977, *Inquiry into Unemployment Benefit Policy and Administration: Report*, Canberra: AGPS

Piggott, J., and B. Chapman 1995, 'Costing the Job Compact', *Economic Record*, 71(215): 313–28

Purdon, C. 1993, *Local and Regional Employment Initiatives and their Co-ordination*, Consultant's report prepared for the Taskforce on Employment Opportunities

Quiggin, J. 1993, 'A Policy Program for Full Employment', *Australian Economic Review*, 2nd Quarter: 41–7

Quiggin, J., and J. Langmore 1994, *Work For All: Full Employment in the Nineties*, Melbourne: Melbourne University Press

Singleton, G. 1994, 'Political Review April–June 1994', *Australian Quarterly*, 66(1): 97–110

Stilwell, F. 1994, '*Working Nation:* From Green Paper to White Paper', in *Journal of Australian Political Economy*, 33: 110–23

Stromback, T. and A. M. Dockery 1998, 'The Job Compact Mark II', *Economic Papers*, 17(2): 24–34

CONCLUDING OBSERVATIONS

Dalton, T., M. Draper, W. Weeks and J. Wiseman 1996, *Making Social Policy in Australia: An Introduction*, Sydney: Allen & Unwin

Edwards M. 1996, Lessons from Prime Minister and the Cabinet', in J. Uhr and K. Mackay (eds), *Evaluating Policy Advice*, Canberra: Federalism Research Centre and ANU, pp. 73–82

Glenn G. G. 1993, 'The Development of the 1992–93 Carers Package: Summary of a Policy Management Review prepared for the Department of Prime Minister and Cabinet', April

Howard, C. 1998, *Carrots and Sticks; A Means Testing State Changes its Mind*, unpublished dissertation, Griffith University

Keating, M. 1994, 'The Role of Government Economists', 1994 Higgins Memorial Lecture, reprinted in *Canberra Bulletin of Public Administration*, 77(2): 1–7

Kingdon, J. W. 1984, *Agendas, Alternatives and Public Policies*, Boston: Little, Brown & Co.

Painter, M., and B. Carey 1979, *Politics Between Departments*, Brisbane: University of Queensland Press

Podger, A. 2000, 'Policy Learning and Health', *Australian Journal of Public Administration*, 59(1): 127–8

Waller M. 1992, 'Evaluating Policy Advice', *Australian Journal of Public Administration*, 51(4): 440–6

Weller, P. 1995, 'Commonwealth–State Reform Processes: A Policy Management Review prepared for the Department of the Prime Minister and Cabinet', June

Index

Printed and bound by CPI Group (UK) Ltd, Croydon, CR0 4YY

23/10/2024

01777665-0007